Lippincott's Photo Atlas of Medication Administration

Fourth Edition

Pamela Lynn, MSN, RN
Instructor
School of Nursing
Gwynedd-Mercy College
Gwynedd Valley, Pennsylvania

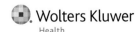 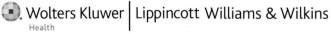

Health

Philadelphia · Baltimore · New York · London
Buenos Aires · Hong Kong · Sydney · Tokyo

Executive Acquisitions Editor: Hilarie Surrena
Product Managers: Helene T. Caprari
Design Coordinator: Holly Reid McLaughlin
Art Director, Illustration: Brett MacNaughton
Manufacturing Coordinator: Karin Duffield
Prepress Vendor: Aptara, Inc.

Fourth Edition

9 8 7 6 5 4

Printed in China

ISBN: 9781451112481

Care has been taken to confirm the accuracy of the information presented and to describe generally accepted practices. However, the author, editors, and publisher are not responsible for errors or omissions or for any consequences from application of the information in this book and make no warranty, expressed or implied, with respect to the currency, completeness, or accuracy of the contents of the publication. Application of this information in a particular situation remains the professional responsibility of the practitioner; the clinical treatments described and recommended may not be considered absolute and universal recommendations.

The author, editors, and publisher have exerted every effort to ensure that drug selection and dosage set forth in this text are in accordance with the current recommendations and practice at the time of publication. However, in view of ongoing research, changes in government regulations, and the constant flow of information relating to drug therapy and drug reactions, the reader is urged to check the package insert for each drug for any change in indications and dosage and for added warnings and precautions. This is particularly important when the recommended agent is a new or infrequently employed drug.

Some drugs and medical devices presented in this publication have US Food and Drug Administration (FDA) clearance for limited use in restricted research settings. It is the responsibility of the healthcare provider to ascertain the FDA status of each drug or device planned for use in his or her clinical practice.

LWW.com

Contents

Skill · 1   Administering Oral Medications

Drugs given orally are intended for absorption in the stomach and small intestine. The oral route is the most commonly used route of administration. It is usually the most convenient and comfortable route for the patient. After oral administration, drug action has a slower onset and a more prolonged, but less potent, effect than other routes.

EQUIPMENT

- Medication in disposable cup or oral syringe
- Liquid (e.g., water, juice) with straw, if not contraindicated
- Medication cart or tray
- Computer-generated Medication Administration Record (CMAR) or Medication Administration Record (MAR)
- PPE, as indicated

ASSESSMENT

Assess the appropriateness of the drug for the patient. Review medical history, allergy, assessment, and laboratory data that may influence drug administration. Assess the patient's ability to swallow medications. If the patient cannot swallow, is NPO, or is experiencing nausea or vomiting, withhold the medication, notify the primary care provider, and complete proper documentation. Assess the patient's knowledge of the medication. If the patient has a knowledge deficit about the medication, this may be the appropriate time to begin education about the medication. If the medication may affect the patient's vital signs, assess them before administration. If the medication is for pain relief, assess the patient's pain level before and after administration. Verify the patient name, dose, route, and time of administration.

NURSING DIAGNOSIS

Determine related factors for the nursing diagnoses based on the patient's current status. Appropriate nursing diagnoses may include:
- Impaired Swallowing
- Deficient Knowledge
- Noncompliance
- Risk for Aspiration
- Anxiety

OUTCOME IDENTIFICATION AND PLANNING

The expected outcome to achieve when administering an oral medication is that the patient will swallow the medication. Other outcomes that may be appropriate include the following: the patient will experience the desired effect from the medication; the patient will not aspirate; the patient experiences decreased anxiety; the patient does not experience adverse effects; and the patient understands and complies with the medication regimen.

IMPLEMENTATION

ACTION	RATIONALE
1. Gather equipment. Check each medication order against the original in the medical record, according to facility policy. Clarify any inconsistencies. Check the patient's chart for allergies.	This comparison helps to identify errors that may have occurred when orders were transcribed. The primary care provider's order is the legal record of medication orders for each facility.
2. Know the actions, special nursing considerations, safe dose ranges, purpose of administration, and adverse effects of the medications to be administered. Consider the appropriateness of the medication for this patient.	This knowledge aids the nurse in evaluating the therapeutic effect of the medication in relation to the patient's disorder and can also be used to educate the patient about the medication.
3. Perform hand hygiene.	Hand hygiene prevents the spread of microorganisms.
4. Move the medication cart to the outside of the patient's room or prepare for administration in the medication area.	Organization facilitates error-free administration and saves time.
5. Unlock the medication cart or drawer. Enter pass code into the computer and scan employee identification, if required.	Locking the cart or drawer safeguards each patient's medication supply. Hospital accrediting organizations require medication carts to be locked when not in use. Entering pass code and scanning ID allows only authorized users into the computer system and identifies the user for documentation by the computer.

(continued)

Skill · 1   Administering Oral Medications   *continued*

ACTION

6. **Prepare medications for one patient at a time.**

7. Read the CMAR/MAR and select the proper medication from the patient's medication drawer or unit stock.

8. Compare the label with the CMAR/MAR (Figure 1). Check expiration dates and perform calculations, if necessary. Scan the bar code on the package, if required.

9. Prepare the required medications:

    a. *Unit dose packages:* Place unit dose-packaged medications in a disposable cup. **Do not open the wrapper until at the bedside.** Keep narcotics and medications that require special nursing assessments in a separate container.

    b. *Multidose containers:* When removing tablets or capsules from a multidose bottle, pour the necessary number into the bottle cap and then place the tablets or capsules in a medication cup. Break only scored tablets, if necessary, to obtain the proper dosage. Do not touch tablets or capsules with hands.

    c. *Liquid medication in multidose bottle:* When pouring liquid medications out of a multidose bottle, hold the bottle so the label is against the palm. Use the appropriate measuring device when pouring liquids, and read the amount of medication at the bottom of the meniscus at eye level (Figure 2). Wipe the lip of the bottle with a paper towel.

RATIONALE

This prevents errors in medication administration.

This is the *first* check of the label.

This is the *second* check of the label. Verify calculations with another nurse to ensure safety, if necessary.

Wrapper is kept intact because the label is needed for an additional safety check. Special assessments may be required before giving certain medications. These may include assessing vital signs and checking laboratory test results.

Pouring medication into the cap allows for easy return of excess medication to the bottle. Pouring tablets or capsules your hand is unsanitary.

Liquid that may drip onto the label makes the label difficult to read. Accuracy is possible when the appropriate measuring device is used and then read accurately.

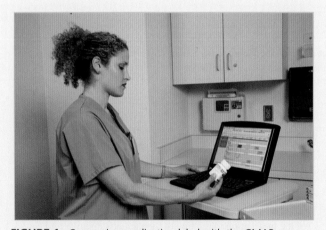

FIGURE 1. Comparing medication label with the CMAR.

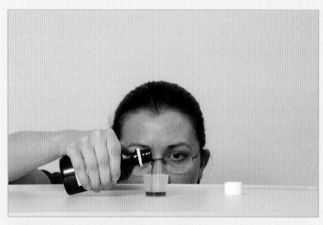

FIGURE 2. Measuring at eye level. *(Photo by B. Proud.)*

10. **When all medications for one patient have been prepared, recheck the labels with the CMAR/MAR before taking the medications to the patient. Replace any multidose containers in the patient's drawer or unit stock. Lock the medication cart before leaving it.**

11. Transport medications to the patient's bedside carefully, and keep the medications in sight at all times.

12. **Ensure that the patient receives the medications at the correct time.**

This is a *third* check to ensure accuracy and to prevent errors. Locking the cart or drawer safeguards the patient's medication supply. Hospital accrediting organizations require medication carts to be locked when not in use. Some facilities require the third check to occur at the bedside, after identifying the patient and before administration.

Careful handling and close observation prevent accidental or deliberate disarrangement of medications.

Check agency policy, which may allow for administration within a period of 30 minutes before or 30 minutes after the designated time.

ACTION	RATIONALE

13. Perform hand hygiene and put on PPE, if indicated.

Hand hygiene and PPE prevent the spread of microorganisms. PPE is required based on transmission precautions.

14. Identify the patient. Usually, the patient should be identified using two methods. Compare the information with the CMAR/MAR.

Identifying the patient ensures that the right patient receives the medications and helps prevent errors.

   a. Check the name and identification number on the patient's identification band (Figure 3).

This is the most reliable method. Replace the identification band if it is missing or inaccurate in any way.

   b. Ask the patient to state his or her name and birth date, based on facility policy.

This requires a response from the patient, but illness and strange surroundings often cause patients to be confused.

   c. If the patient cannot identify him- or herself, verify the patient's identification with a staff member who knows the patient, for the second source.

This is another way to double check identity. Do not use the name on the door or over the bed, because these signs may be inaccurate.

15. **Scan the patient's bar code on the identification band, if required (Figure 4).**

The bar code provides an additional check to ensure that the medication is given to the right patient.

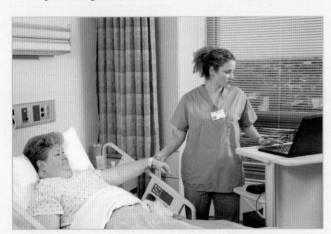

FIGURE 3. Comparing patient's name and identification number with the CMAR.

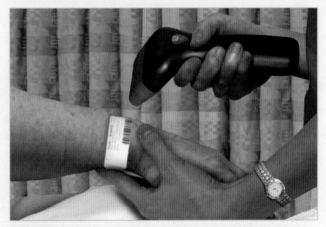

FIGURE 4. Scanning the bar code on the patient's identification bracelet. *(Photo by B. Proud.)*

16. **Complete necessary assessments before administering medications. Check the patient's allergy bracelet or ask the patient about allergies. Explain the purpose and action of each medication to the patient.**

Assessment is a prerequisite to administration of medications.

17. Assist the patient to an upright or lateral position.

Swallowing is facilitated by proper positioning. An upright or side-lying position protects the patient from aspiration.

18. Administer medications:

   a. Offer water or other permitted fluids with pills, capsules, tablets, and some liquid medications.

Liquids facilitate swallowing of solid drugs. Some liquid drugs are intended to adhere to the pharyngeal area, in which case liquid is not offered with the medication.

   b. Ask whether the patient prefers to take the medications by hand or in a cup.

This encourages the patient's participation in taking the medications.

19. **Remain with the patient until each medication is swallowed. Never leave medication at the patient's bedside (Figure 5).**

Unless you have seen the patient swallow the drug, the drug cannot be recorded as administered. The patient's chart is a legal record. Only with a physician's order can medications be left at the bedside.

(continued)

Skill · 1   **Administering Oral Medications**   *continued*

ACTION

RATIONALE

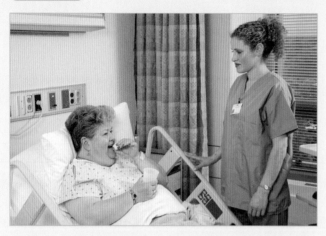

FIGURE 5. Remaining with the patient until each medication is swallowed.

20. Assist the patient to a comfortable position. Remove PPE, if used. Perform hand hygiene.

Promotes patient comfort. Proper removal of PPE prevents transmission of microorganisms. Hand hygiene deters the spread of microorganisms.

21. Document the administration of the medication immediately after administration. See Documentation section below.

Timely documentation helps to ensure patient safety.

22. Evaluate the patient's response to medication within appropriate time frame.

The patient needs to be evaluated for therapeutic and adverse effects from the medication.

EVALUATION

The expected outcomes are met when the patient swallows the medication, does not aspirate, verbalizes an understanding of the medication, experiences the desired effect from the medication, and does not experience adverse effects.

DOCUMENTATION

Guidelines

Record each medication administered on the CMAR/MAR or record using the required format immediately after it is administered, including date and time of administration (Figure 6). If using a bar-code system, medication administration is automatically recorded when the bar code is scanned. PRN medications require documentation of the reason for administration. Prompt recording avoids the possibility of accidentally repeating the administration of the drug. If the drug was refused or omitted, record this in the appropriate area on the medication record and notify the primary care provider. This verifies the reason medication was omitted and ensures that the primary care provider is aware of the patient's condition. Recording administration of a narcotic may require additional documentation on a narcotic record, stating drug count and other specific information. A record of fluid intake and output measurement is required.

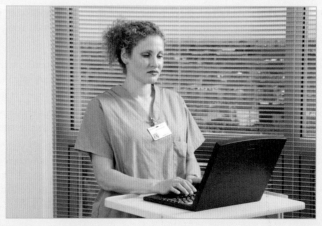

FIGURE 6. Recording each medication administered on the CMAR.

> 8/6/12 0835 Patient states he is having constant stabbing leg pains. Rates pain as an 8/10. Percocet 2 tabs administered.
>
> —*K. Sanders, RN*
>
> 8/6/12 0905 Patient resting comfortably. Rates leg pain as a 1/10.
>
> —*K. Sanders, RN*
>
> 8/6/12 1300 Patient states he does not want pain medication, despite return of leg pain. States, "It made me feel woozy last time." Feelings discussed with patient. Patient agrees to take Percocet 1 tab at this time.
>
> —*K. Sanders, RN*
>
> 8/6/12 1320 Percocet, 1 tablet given PO.
>
> —*K. Sanders, RN*

UNEXPECTED SITUATIONS AND ASSOCIATED INTERVENTIONS

- *Patient states that it feels like medication is lodged in throat:* Offer patient more fluids to drink. If allowed, offer the patient bread or crackers to help move the medication to the stomach.
- *It is unclear whether the patient swallowed the medication:* Check in the patient's mouth, under tongue, and between cheek and gum. Patients with altered mental status may not be aware that the medication was not swallowed. Also, patients may "cheek" medications to avoid taking the medication or to save it for later use. Watch patients requiring suicide precautions closely to ensure that they are not "cheeking" the medication or hiding it in the mouth. These patients may be trying to accumulate a large amount of medication to take all at once in a suicide attempt. Substance abusers may cheek medication to accumulate a large amount to take all at once so that they may feel a high from medication.
- *Patient vomits immediately or shortly after receiving oral medication:* Assess vomit, looking for pills or fragments. Do not readminister medication without notifying primary care provider. If a whole pill is seen and can be identified, the primary care provider may ask that the medication be administered again. If a pill is not seen or medications cannot be identified, do not readminister the medication in order to prevent the patient from receiving too large a dose.
- *Child refuses to take oral medications:* Some medications may be mixed in a small amount of food, such as pudding or ice cream. Do not add the medication to liquids because the medication may alter the taste of liquids; if child then refuses to drink the rest of the liquid, you will not know how much of the medication was ingested. Use creativity when devising ways to administer medications to a child. See the section below, Infant and Child Considerations, for suggestions.
- *The capsule or tablet falls to the floor during administration.* Discard and obtain a new dose for administration. This prevents contamination and transmission of microorganisms.
- *Patient refuses medication.* Explore the reason for the patient's refusal. Review the rationale for using the drug and any other information that may be appropriate. If you are unable to administer the medication despite education and discussion, document the omission according to facility policy and notify the primary care provider.

SPECIAL CONSIDERATIONS
General Considerations

- Some liquid medication preparations, such as suspensions, require agitation to ensure even distribution of medication in the solution. Be familiar with the specific requirements for medications you are administering.
- Place medications intended for sublingual absorption under the patient's tongue. Instruct the patient to allow the medication to dissolve completely. Reinforce the importance of not swallowing the medication tablet.
- Some oral medications are provided in powdered forms. Verify the correct liquid to dissolve the medication in for administration. This information is usually included on the package; verify any unclear instructions with a pharmacist or medication reference. If there is more than one possible liquid to dissolve the medication in, include the patient in the decision process; patients may find one choice more palatable than another.

(continued)

- Ongoing assessment is an important part of nursing care for both evaluation of patient response to administered medications and early detection of adverse effects. If an adverse effect is suspected, withhold further medication doses and notify the patient's primary care provider. Additional intervention is based on type of reaction and patient assessment.
- If the patient questions a medication order or states the medication is different from the usual dose, always recheck and clarify with the original order and/or primary care provider before giving the medication.
- If the patient's level of consciousness is altered or his or her swallowing is impaired, check with the primary care provider to clarify the route of administration or alternative forms of medication. This may also be a solution for a pediatric or a confused patient who is refusing to take a medication.
- Patients with poor vision can request large-type labels on medication containers. A magnifying lens also may be helpful.
- Provide written medication information to reinforce discussion and education in the appropriate language, if the patient is literate. If the patient is unable to read, provide written information to family or significant other, if appropriate. Written information should be at a 5th-grade level to ensure ease of understanding.
- If the patient has difficulty swallowing tablets, it may be appropriate to crush the medication to facilitate administration. However, not all medications can be crushed or altered; long-acting and slow-release drugs are examples of medications that cannot be crushed. Therefore, it is important to consult a medication reference and/or pharmacist. If the medication can be crushed, use a pill-crusher or mortar and pestle to grind the tablet into a powder. Crush each pill one at a time. Dissolve the powder with water or other recommended liquid in a liquid medication cup, keeping each medication separate from the others. Keep the package label with the medication cup for future comparison of information. Combine the crushed medication with a small amount of soft food, such as applesauce or pudding, to facilitate administration.

Infant and Child Considerations

- Special devices, such as oral syringes and calibrated nipples, are available in a pharmacy to ensure accurate dose calculations for young children and infants.
- Some creative ways to administer medications to children include the following: have a "tea party" with medicine cups; place oral syringe (without needle) or dropper in the space between the cheek and gum and slowly administer the medication; save a special treat for after the medication administration (e.g., movie, playroom time, or a special food, if allowed).
- The FDA has received reports of infants choking on the plastic caps that fit on the end of syringes when used to administer oral medications. They recommend the following: remove and dispose of caps before giving syringes to patients or families, caution family caregivers to dispose of caps on syringes they buy over the counter, and report any problems with syringe caps to the FDA. Companies manufacture syringes labeled "oral use" without the caps on them.

Older Adult Considerations

- Elderly patients with arthritis may have difficulty opening childproof caps. On request, the pharmacist can substitute a cap that is easier to open. A rubber band twisted around the cap may provide a more secure grip for older patients.
- Consider large-print written information, when appropriate.
- Physiologic changes associated with the aging process, including decreased gastric motility, muscle mass, acid production, and blood flow, can affect patient's response to medication, including drug absorption and increased risk of adverse effects. Older adults are more likely to take multiple drugs, so drug interactions in the older adult are a very real and dangerous problem. Refer to Fundamentals Review 5-6.

Home Care Considerations

- Encourage the patient to discard expired prescription medications.
- Discuss safe storage of medications when there are children and pets in the environment.
- Discuss with parents the difference in over-the-counter medications made for infants and medications made for children. Many times parents do not realize that there are different strengths to the actual medications, leading to under- or overdosing.
- Encourage patients to carry a card listing all medications, dosage, and frequency in case of an emergency.
- Discuss the importance of using an appropriate measuring device for liquid medications. Caution patients not to use eating utensils for measuring medications; use a liquid medication cup, oral syringe, or measuring spoon to provide accurate dosing.

Skill · 2   Administering Medications via a Gastric Tube

Patients with a gastrointestinal tube (nasogastric, nasointestinal, percutaneous endoscopic gastrostomy [PEG], or jejunostomy [J] tube) often receive medication through the tube. Care of the patient with an enteral feeding tube is described in Chapter 11, Nutrition. Use liquid medications, when possible, because they are readily absorbed and less likely to cause tube occlusions. Certain solid dosage medications can be crushed and combined with liquid. Medications should be crushed to a fine powder and mixed with 15 to 30 mL of water before delivery through the tube. Certain capsules may be opened, emptied into liquid, and administered through the tube (Toedter Williams, 2008). Check manufacturer's recommendations and/or with a pharmacist to verify.

EQUIPMENT

- Irrigation set (60-mL syringe and irrigation container)
- Medications
- Water (gastrostomy tubes) or sterile water (nasogastric tubes), according to facility policy
- Gloves
- Additional PPE, as indicated

ASSESSMENT

Research each medication to be given, especially for mode of action, side effects, nursing implications, ability to be crushed, and whether the medication should be given with or without food. Verify patient name, dose, route, and time of administration. Also assess patient's knowledge of medication and the reason for its administration. Auscultate the abdomen for evidence of bowel sounds. Percuss and palpate the abdomen for tenderness and distention. Ascertain the time of the patient's last bowel movement and measure abdominal girth, if appropriate.

NURSING DIAGNOSIS

Determine the related factors for the nursing diagnoses based on the patient's current status. Possible nursing diagnoses may include:
- Deficient Knowledge
- Risk for Injury
- Impaired Swallowing

OUTCOME IDENTIFICATION AND PLANNING

The expected outcome to achieve is that the patient receives the medication via the tube and experiences the intended effect of the medication. In addition, the patient verbalizes knowledge of the medications given; the patient remains free from adverse effect and injury; and the gastrointestinal tube remains patent.

IMPLEMENTATION

ACTION	RATIONALE
1. Gather equipment. Check each medication order against the original in the medical record, according to facility policy. Clarify any inconsistencies. Check the patient's chart for allergies.	This comparison helps to identify errors that may have occurred when orders were transcribed. The primary care provider's order is the legal record of medication orders for each facility.
2. Know the actions, special nursing considerations, safe dose ranges, purpose of administration, and adverse effects of the medications to be administered. Consider the appropriateness of the medication for this patient.	This knowledge aids the nurse in evaluating the therapeutic effect of the medication in relation to the patient's disorder and can also be used to educate the patient about the medication.
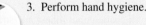 3. Perform hand hygiene.	Hand hygiene prevents the spread of microorganisms.
4. Move the medication cart to the outside of the patient's room or prepare for administration in the medication area.	Organization facilitates error-free administration and saves time.
5. Unlock the medication cart or drawer. Enter pass code and scan employee identification, if required.	Locking the cart or drawer safeguards each patient's medication supply. Hospital accrediting organizations require medication carts to be locked when not in use. Entering pass code and scanning ID allows only authorized users into the system and identifies user for documentation by the computer.
6. **Prepare medications for one patient at a time.**	This prevents errors in medication administration.

(continued)

Skill · 2   Administering Medications via a Gastric Tube   *continued*

ACTION	RATIONALE
7. Read the CMAR/MAR and select the proper medication from the patient's medication drawer or unit stock.	This is the *first* check of the label.
8. Compare the label with the CMAR/MAR. Check expiration dates and perform calculations, if necessary. Scan the bar code on the package, if required.	This is the *second* check of the label. Verify calculations with another nurse to ensure safety, if necessary.
9. Check to see if medications to be administered come in a liquid form. **If pills or capsules are to be given, check with pharmacy or drug reference to verify the ability to crush or open capsules.**	To prevent the tube from becoming clogged, all medications should be given in liquid form whenever possible. Medications in extended-release formulations should not be crushed before administration.
10. Prepare medication.	
Pills: Using a pill crusher, crush each pill one at a time. Dissolve the powder with water or other recommended liquid in a liquid medication cup, keeping each medication separate from the others. Keep the package label with the medication cup, for future comparison of information.	Some medications require dissolution in liquid other than water. The label is needed for an additional safety check. Some medications require pre-administration assessments.
Liquid: When pouring liquid medications from a multidose bottle, hold the bottle with the label against the palm. Use the appropriate measuring device when pouring liquids, and read the amount of medication at the bottom of the meniscus at eye level. Wipe the lip of the bottle with a paper towel.	Liquid that may drip onto the label makes the label difficult to read. Accuracy is possible when the appropriate measuring device is used and then read accurately.
11. **When all medications for one patient have been prepared, recheck the label with the MAR before taking the medications to the patient.**	This is a *third* check to ensure accuracy and to prevent errors. Some facilities require the third check to occur at the bedside, after identifying the patient and before administration.
12. Lock the medication cart before leaving it.	Locking the cart or drawer safeguards the patient's medication supply. Hospital accrediting organizations require medication carts to be locked when not in use.
13. Transport medications to the patient's bedside carefully, and keep the medications in sight at all times.	Careful handling and close observation prevent accidental or deliberate disarrangement of medications.
14. **Ensure that the patient receives the medications at the correct time.**	Check agency policy, which may allow for administration within a period of 30 minutes before or 30 minutes after designated time.
15. Perform hand hygiene and put on PPE, if indicated.	Hand hygiene and PPE prevent the spread of microorganisms. PPE is required based on transmission precautions.
16. Identify the patient. Usually, the patient should be identified using two methods. Compare information with the CMAR/MAR.	Identifying the patient ensures the right patient receives the medications and helps prevent errors.
a. Check the name and identification number on the patient's identification band.	This is the most reliable method. Replace the identification band if it is missing or inaccurate in any way.
b. Ask the patient to state his or her name and birth date, based on facility policy.	This requires a response from the patient, but illness and strange surroundings often cause patients to be confused.
c. If the patient cannot identify him- or herself, verify the patient's identification with a staff member who knows the patient for the second source.	This is another way to double-check identity. Do not use the name on the door or over the bed, because these signs may be inaccurate.
17. Complete necessary assessments before administering medications. Check the patient's allergy bracelet or ask the patient about allergies. Explain what you are going to do, and the reason for doing it, to the patient.	Assessment is a prerequisite to administration of medications. Explanation relieves anxiety and facilitates cooperation.
18. Scan the patient's bar code on the identification band, if required.	This provides an additional check to ensure that the medication is given to the right patient.

| ACTION | RATIONALE |

19. Assist the patient to the high Fowler's position, unless contraindicated.

This reduces the risk of aspiration.

20. Put on gloves.

Gloves prevent contact with mucous membranes and body fluids.

21. If patient is receiving continuous tube feedings, pause the tube-feeding pump (Figure 1).

If the pump is not stopped, tube feeding will flow out of the tube and onto the patient.

22. Pour the water into the irrigation container. Measure 30 mL of water. Apply clamp on feeding tube, if present. Alternately, pinch gastric tube below port with fingers, or position stopcock to correct direction. Open port on gastric tube delegated to medication administration (Figure 2) or disconnect tubing for feeding from gastric tube and place cap on end of feeding tubing.

Fluid is ready for flushing of the tube. Applying clamp, folding the tube over and clamping, or the correct positioning of the stopcock prevents any backflow of gastric drainage. Covering end of feeding tubing prevents contamination.

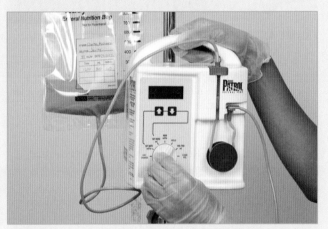

FIGURE 1. Pausing feeding pump. *(Photo by B. Proud.)*

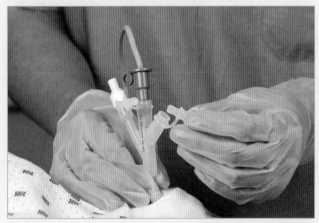

FIGURE 2. Pinching gastric tubing to prevent backflow of gastric drainage and opening medication administration port. *(Photo by B. Proud.)*

23. **Check placement of tube, depending on type of tube and facility policy.** (Refer to Chapter 11, Nutrition.)

Tube placement must be confirmed before administering anything through the tube to avoid inadvertent instillation in the respiratory tract.

24. Note the amount of any residual. Refer to Chapter 11, Nutrition. Replace residual back into stomach, based on facility policy.

Research findings are inconclusive on the benefit of returning gastric volumes to the stomach or intestine to avoid fluid or electrolyte imbalance, which has been accepted practice. Consult agency policy concerning this practice (Bourgault, et al., 2007; Keithley & Swanson, 2004; Metheny, 2008).

25. Apply clamp on feeding tube, if present. Alternately, pinch gastric tube below port with fingers, or position stopcock to correct direction. Remove 60-mL syringe gastric tube. Remove the plunger of the syringe. Reinsert the syringe in the gastric tube without the plunger. Pour 30 mL of water into the syringe (Figure 3). **Unclamp the tube and allow the water to enter the stomach via gravity infusion.**

Folding the tube over and clamping it prevents any backflow of gastric drainage. Flushing the tube ensures all the residual is cleared from tube.

26. Administer the first dose of medication by pouring into the syringe (Figure 4). Follow with a 5- to 10-mL water flush between medication doses. Follow the last dose of medication with 30 to 60 mL of water flush.

Flushing between medications prevents any possible interactions between the medications. Flushing at the end maintains patency of the tube, prevents blockage by medication particles, and ensures all doses enter the stomach.

(continued)

Skill · 2 Administering Medications via a Gastric Tube *continued*

ACTION

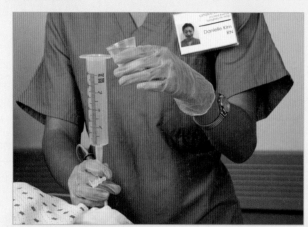

FIGURE 3. Pouring water into syringe inserted in gastric tube. *(Photo by B. Proud.)*

27. Clamp the tube, remove the syringe, and replace the feeding tubing. If stopcock is used, position stopcock to correct direction. If tube medication port was used, cap port. Unclamp gastric tube and restart tube feeding, if appropriate for medications administered.

28. Remove gloves. Assist the patient to a comfortable position. If receiving a tube feeding, the head of the bed must remain elevated at least 30 degrees.

 29. Remove additional PPE, if used. Perform hand hygiene.

30. Document the administration of the medication immediately after administration. See Documentation section below.

31. Evaluate the patient's response to medication within appropriate time frame.

RATIONALE

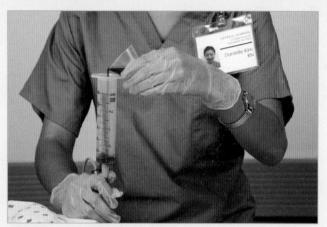

FIGURE 4. Pouring medication into syringe inserted in gastric tube. *(Photo by B. Proud.)*

Some medications require the holding of the tube feeding for a certain period of time after administration. Consult a drug reference or a pharmacist.

Ensures patient comfort. Keeping the head of the bed elevated helps prevent aspiration.

Removing PPE properly reduces the risk for infection transmission and contamination of other items. Hand hygiene prevents the spread of microorganisms.

Timely documentation helps to ensure patient safety.

The patient needs to be evaluated for therapeutic and adverse effects from the medication.

EVALUATION

The expected outcome is met when the patient receives the ordered medications and experiences the intended effects of the medications administered. In addition, the patient demonstrates a patent and functioning gastric tube, verbalizes knowledge of the medications given, and remains free from adverse effect and injury.

DOCUMENTATION
Guidelines

Document the administration of the medication immediately after administration, including date, time, dose, and route of administration on the CMAR/MAR or record using the required format. If using a bar-code system, medication administration is automatically recorded when the bar code is scanned. PRN medications require documentation of the reason for administration. Prompt recording avoids the possibility of accidentally repeating the administration of the drug. Record the amount of gastric residual, if appropriate. Record the amount of liquid given on the intake and output record. If the drug was refused or omitted, record this in the appropriate area on the medication record and notify the primary care provider. This verifies the reason medication was omitted and ensures that the primary care provider is aware of the patient's condition.

UNEXPECTED SITUATIONS AND ASSOCIATED INTERVENTIONS

• *Medication enters tube and then tube becomes clogged:* Attach a 10-mL syringe onto end of tube. Pull back and then lightly apply pressure to plunger in a repetitive motion. This may dislodge the medication. If the medication does not move through the tube, notify the primary care provider. The tube may have to be replaced.

SPECIAL CONSIDERATIONS

- If medications are being administered via an NG tube that is attached to suction, the tube should remain clamped, off suction, for a period of time after medication administration. This allows for medication absorption before returning to suction. Check facility policy and drug reference for specific drug requirements.
- If necessary to use plunger in irrigation syringe to administer medications, instill gently and slowly. Gravity administration is considered best to avoid excess pressure.
- Give medications separately and flush with water between each drug. Some medications may interact with each other or become less effective if mixed with other drugs.
- If the patient is receiving tube feedings, review information about the drugs to be administered. Absorption of some drugs, such as phenytoin (Dilantin), is affected by tube feeding formulas. Discontinue a continuous tube feeding and leave the tube clamped for the required period of time before and after the medication has been given, according to the reference and facility protocol.
- Ongoing assessment is an important part of nursing care for both evaluation of patient response to administered medications and early detection of adverse effects. If an adverse effect is suspected, withhold further medication doses and notify the patient's primary healthcare provider. Additional intervention is based on type of reaction and patient assessment.

Skill · 3   Removing Medication from an Ampule

An ampule is a glass flask that contains a single dose of medication for parenteral administration. Because there is no way to prevent contamination of any unused portion of medication after the ampule is opened, if not all the medication is used, discard any remaining medication. Remove medication from an ampule after its thin neck is broken.

EQUIPMENT

- Sterile syringe and filter needle
- Ampule of medication
- Small gauze pad
- Computer-generated Medication Administration Record (CMAR) or Medication Administration Record (MAR)

ASSESSMENT

Assess the medication in the ampule for any particles or discoloration. Assess the ampule for any cracks or chips. Check expiration date before administering the medication. Verify patient name, dose, route, and time of administration. Assess the appropriateness of the drug for the patient. Review assessment and laboratory data that may influence drug administration.

NURSING DIAGNOSIS

Determine related factors for the nursing diagnoses based on the patient's current status. Appropriate nursing diagnoses may include:

- Risk for Infection
- Anxiety
- Deficient Knowledge
- Risk for Injury

OUTCOME IDENTIFICATION AND PLANNING

The expected outcome to achieve when removing medication from an ampule is that the medication will be removed in a sterile manner; it will be free from glass shards and the proper dose prepared.

IMPLEMENTATION

ACTION	RATIONALE
1. Gather equipment. Check the medication order against the original order in the medical record, according to facility policy. Clarify any inconsistencies. Check the patient's chart for allergies.	This comparison helps to identify errors that may have occurred when orders were transcribed. The primary care provider's order is the legal record of medication orders for each facility.

(continued)

Skill · 3 Removing Medication from an Ampule *continued*

ACTION

2. Know the actions, special nursing considerations, safe dose ranges, purpose of administration, and adverse effects of the medications to be administered. Consider the appropriateness of the medication for this patient.

    3. Perform hand hygiene.

4. Move the medication cart to the outside of the patient's room or prepare for administration in the medication area.

5. Unlock the medication cart or drawer. Enter pass code and scan employee identification, if required.

6. **Prepare medications for one patient at a time.**

7. Read the CMAR/MAR and select the proper medication from the patient's medication drawer or unit stock.

8. Compare the label with the CMAR/MAR. Check expiration dates and perform calculations, if necessary. Scan the bar code on the package, if required.

9. Tap the stem of the **ampule** (Figure 1) or twist your wrist quickly (Figure 2) while holding the ampule vertically.

RATIONALE

This knowledge aids the nurse in evaluating the therapeutic effect of the medication in relation to the patient's disorder and can also be used to educate the patient about the medication.

Hand hygiene deters the spread of microorganisms.

Organization facilitates error-free administration and saves time.

Locking the cart or drawer safeguards each patient's medication supply. Hospital accrediting organizations require medication carts to be locked when not in use. Entering pass code and scanning ID allows only authorized users into the system and identifies user for documentation by the computer.

This prevents errors in medication administration.

This is the *first* check of the label.

This is the *second* check of the label. Verify calculations with another nurse to ensure safety, if necessary.

This facilitates movement of medication in the stem to the body of the ampule.

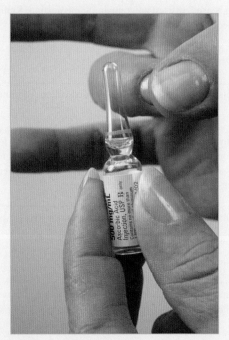

FIGURE 1. Tapping stem of the ampule.

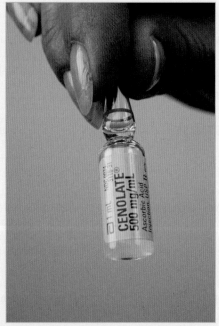

FIGURE 2. Twisting wrist quickly while holding the ampule vertically.

10. Wrap a small gauze pad around the neck of the ampule.

11. Use a snapping motion to break off the top of the ampule along the scored line at its neck (Figure 3). **Always break away from your body.**

This will protect your fingers from the glass as the ampule is broken.

This protects your face and fingers from any shattered glass fragments.

ACTION   RATIONALE

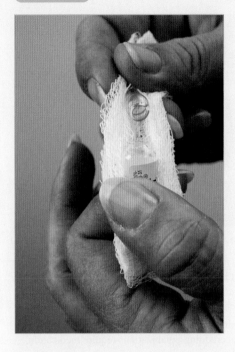

FIGURE 3. Using a snapping motion to break top of the ampule.

12. Attach filter needle to syringe. Remove the cap from the filter needle by pulling it straight off.

Use of a filter needle prevents the accidental withdrawing of small glass particles with the medication. Pulling the cap off in a straight manner prevents accidental needlestick.

13. Withdraw medication in the amount ordered plus a small amount more (approximately 30% more). **Do not inject air into the solution.** Use either of the following methods. **While inserting the filter needle into the ampule, be careful not to touch the rim.**

By withdrawing an additional small amount of medication, any air bubbles in the syringe can be displaced once the syringe is removed and ample medication will still remain in the syringe. The contents of the ampule are not under pressure; therefore, air is unnecessary and will cause the contents to overflow. The rim of the ampule is considered contaminated.

   a. Insert the tip of the needle into the ampule, which is upright on a flat surface, and withdraw fluid into the syringe (Figure 4). **Touch the plunger at the knob only.**

Handling the plunger at the knob only will keep the shaft of the plunger sterile.

   b. Insert the tip of the needle into the ampule and invert the ampule. Keep the needle centered and not touching the sides of the ampule. Withdraw fluid into syringe (Figure 5). **Touch the plunger at the knob only.**

Surface tension holds the fluids in the ampule when inverted. If the needle touches the sides or is removed and then reinserted into the ampule, surface tension is broken, and fluid runs out. Handling the plunger at the knob only will keep the shaft of the plunger sterile.

14. Wait until the needle has been withdrawn to tap the syringe and expel the air carefully by pushing on the plunger. **Check the amount of medication in the syringe with the medication dose and discard any surplus, according to facility policy.**

Ejecting air into the solution increases pressure in the ampule and can force the medication to spill out over the ampule. Ampules may have overfill. Careful measurement ensures that the correct dose is withdrawn.

15. **Recheck the label with the CMAR/MAR.**

This is the *third* check to ensure accuracy and to prevent errors. Some facilities require the third check to occur at the bedside, after identifying the patient and before administration.

16. **Engage safety guard on filter needle and remove the needle. Discard the filter needle in a suitable container. Attach appropriate administration device to syringe.**

The filter needle used to draw up medication should not be used to administer the medication, to prevent any glass shards from entering the patient.

(continued)

Skill · 3   Removing Medication from an Ampule   *continued*

ACTION

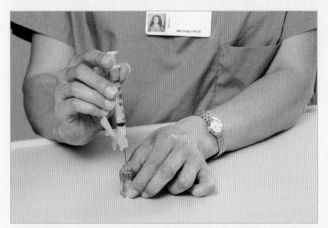

FIGURE 4. Withdrawing medication from upright ampule.

17. Discard the ampule in a suitable container.

18. Lock the medication cart before leaving it.

   19. Perform hand hygiene.

20. Proceed with administration, based on prescribed route.

RATIONALE

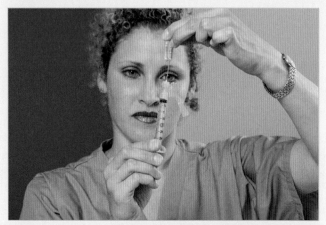

FIGURE 5. Withdrawing medication from inverted ampule.

Any medication that has not been removed from the ampule must be discarded because there is no way to maintain sterility of contents in an opened ampule.

Locking the cart or drawer safeguards the patient's medication supply. Hospital accrediting organizations require medication carts to be locked when not in use.

Hand hygiene deters the spread of microorganisms.

See appropriate skill for prescribed route.

EVALUATION

The expected outcome is met when the medication is removed from the ampule in a sterile manner, free from glass shards, and the proper dose is prepared.

DOCUMENTATION

Guidelines

It is not necessary to record the removal of the medication from the ampule. Record each medication administered on the CMAR/MAR or record using the required format immediately after it is administered, including date and time of administration. If using a bar-code system, medication administration is automatically recorded when the bar code is scanned. PRN medications require documentation of the reason for administration. Prompt recording avoids the possibility of accidentally repeating the administration of the drug. If the drug was refused or omitted, record this in the appropriate area on the medication record and notify the primary care provider. This verifies the reason medication was omitted and ensures that the primary care provider is aware of the patient's condition. Recording administration of a narcotic may require additional documentation on a narcotic record, stating drug count and other specific information. Record fluid intake if intake and output measurement is required.

UNEXPECTED SITUATIONS AND ASSOCIATED INTERVENTIONS

• *You cut yourself while trying to open ampule:* Discard ampule in case contamination has occurred. Bandage wound and obtain a new ampule. Report according to facility policy.
• *All of medication was not removed from the stem and insufficient medication remains in body of ampule for dose:* Discard ampule and drawn medication. Obtain a new ampule and start over. Medication in original ampule stem is considered contaminated once neck of ampule has been placed on a nonsterile surface.
• *You inject air into inverted ampule, spraying medication:* Wash hands to remove any medication. If any medication has gotten into eyes, perform eye irrigation. Obtain a new ampule for medication dose. Report injury, if appropriate, according to facility policy.

- *Medication is drawn up without using a filter needle:* Replace needle with a filter needle. Inject the medication through the filter needle into a new syringe and then administer to patient.
- *Plunger becomes contaminated before inserted into ampule:* Discard needle and syringe and start over. If plunger is contaminated after medication is drawn into the syringe, it is not necessary to discard and start over. The contaminated plunger will enter the barrel of the syringe when pushing the medication out and will not contaminate the medication.

Skill · 4   Removing Medication from a Vial

A vial is a glass bottle with a self-sealing stopper through which medication is removed. For safety in transporting and storing, the vial top is usually covered with a soft metal cap that can be removed easily. The self-sealing stopper that is then exposed is the means of entrance into the vial. Single-dose vials are used once, and then discarded, regardless of the amount of the drug that is used from the vial. Multidose vials contain several doses of medication and can be used multiple times. The Centers for Disease Control and Prevention (CDC) recommends that medications packaged as multiuse vials be assigned to a single patient whenever possible. In addition, it is recommended that the top of the vial be cleaned before each entry, as well as the use of a new sterile needle and syringe (CDC, 2008a; CDC, 2008b). The medication contained in a vial can be in liquid or powder form. Powdered forms must be dissolved in an appropriate diluent before administration. The following skill reviews removing liquid medication from a vial. Refer to the accompanying Skill Variation for steps to reconstitute a powdered medication.

EQUIPMENT

- Sterile syringe and needle or blunt cannula (size depends on medication being administered and patient)
- Vial of medication
- Antimicrobial swab
- Second needle (optional)
- Filter needle (optional)
- Computer-generated Medication Administration Record (CMAR) or Medication Administration Record (MAR)

ASSESSMENT

Assess the medication in the vial for any discoloration or particles. Check expiration date before administering medication. Verify patient name, dose, route, and time of administration. Assess the appropriateness of the drug for the patient. Review assessment and laboratory data that may influence drug administration.

NURSING DIAGNOSIS

Determine related factors for the nursing diagnoses based on the patient's current status. Appropriate nursing diagnoses include:

- Risk for Infection
- Deficient Knowledge
- Risk for Injury
- Anxiety

OUTCOME IDENTIFICATION AND PLANNING

The expected outcome to achieve when removing medication from a vial is withdrawal of the medication into a syringe in a sterile manner and that the proper dose is prepared.

IMPLEMENTATION

ACTION	RATIONALE
1. Gather equipment. Check the medication order against the original order in the medical record, according to facility policy.	This comparison helps to identify errors that may have occurred when orders were transcribed. The primary care provider's order is the legal record of medication orders for each facility.

(continued)

Skill · 4   Removing Medication from a Vial   *continued*

ACTION	RATIONALE

2. Know the actions, special nursing considerations, safe dose ranges, purpose of administration, and adverse effects of the medications to be administered. Consider the appropriateness of the medication for this patient.

This knowledge aids the nurse in evaluating the therapeutic effect of the medication in relation to the patient's disorder and can also be used to educate the patient about the medication.

3. Perform hand hygiene.

Hand hygiene deters the spread of microorganisms.

4. Move the medication cart to the outside of the patient's room or prepare for administration in the medication area.

Organization facilitates error-free administration and saves time.

5. Unlock the medication cart or drawer. Enter pass code and scan employee identification, if required.

Locking the cart or drawer safeguards each patient's medication supply. Hospital accrediting organizations require medication carts to be locked when not in use. Entering pass code and scanning ID allows only authorized users into the system and identifies user for documentation by the computer.

6. **Prepare medications for one patient at a time.**

This prevents errors in medication administration.

7. Read the CMAR/MAR and select the proper medication from the patient's medication drawer or unit stock.

This is the *first* check of the label.

8. Compare the label with the CMAR/MAR. Check expiration dates and perform calculations, if necessary. Scan the bar code on the package, if required.

This is the *second* check of the label. Verify calculations with another nurse to ensure safety, if necessary.

9. Remove the metal or plastic cap on the vial that protects the rubber stopper.

Cap needs to be removed to access medication in **vial.**

10. **Swab the rubber top with the antimicrobial swab and allow to dry.**

Antimicrobial swab removes surface bacteria contamination. Allowing the alcohol to dry prevents it from entering the vial on the needle.

11. Remove the cap from the needle or blunt cannula by pulling it straight off. Touch the plunger at the knob only. Draw back an amount of air into the syringe that is equal to the specific dose of medication to be withdrawn. Some facilities require use of a filter needle when withdrawing premixed medication from multidose vials.

Pulling the cap off in a straight manner prevents accidental needle-stick injury. Handling the plunger at the knob only will keep the shaft of the plunger sterile. Because a vial is a sealed container, before fluid is removed, injection of an equal amount of air is required to prevent the formation of a partial vacuum. If not enough air is injected, the negative pressure makes it difficult to withdraw the medication. Using a filter needle prevents any solid material from being withdrawn through the needle.

12. Hold the vial on a flat surface. Pierce the rubber stopper in the center with the needle tip and inject the measured air into the space above the solution (Figure 1). Do not inject air into the solution.

Air bubbled through the solution could result in withdrawal of an inaccurate amount of medication.

13. **Invert the vial. Keep the tip of the needle or blunt cannula below the fluid level (Figure 2).**

This prevents air from being aspirated into the syringe.

14. Hold the vial in one hand and use the other to withdraw the medication. Touch the plunger at the knob only. **Draw up the prescribed amount of medication while holding the syringe vertically and at eye level (Figure 3).**

Handling the plunger at the knob only will keep the shaft of the plunger sterile. Holding the syringe at eye level facilitates accurate reading, and the vertical position makes removal of air bubbles from the syringe easy.

15. If any air bubbles accumulate in the syringe, tap the barrel of the syringe sharply and move the needle past the fluid into the air space to re-inject the air bubble into the vial. Return the needle tip to the solution and continue withdrawal of the medication.

Removal of air bubbles is necessary to ensure accurate dose of medication.

| ACTION | | RATIONALE |

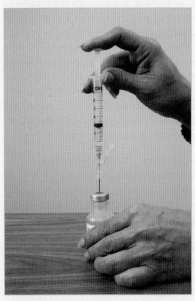

FIGURE 1. Injecting air with vial upright.

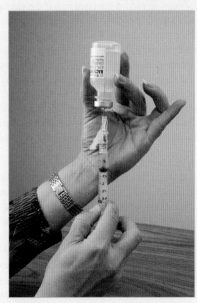

FIGURE 2. Positioning needle tip in solution.

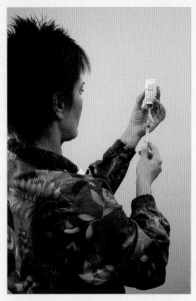

FIGURE 3. Withdrawing medication at eye level.

16. After the correct dose is withdrawn, remove the needle from the vial and carefully replace the cap over the needle. **If a filter needle has been used to draw up the medication, remove it and attach the appropriate administration device.** Some facilities require changing the needle, if one was used to withdraw the medication, before administering the medication.

This prevents contamination of the needle and protects against accidental needlesticks. A one-handed recap method may be used as long as care is taken not to contaminate the needle during the process. A filter needle used to draw up medication should not be used to administer the medication to prevent any solid material from entering the patient. Changing the needle may be necessary because passing the needle through the stopper on the vial may dull the needle.

17. **Check the amount of medication in the syringe with the medication dose and discard any surplus.**

Careful measurement ensures that correct dose is withdrawn.

18. **Recheck the label with the CMAR/MAR.**

This is the *third* check to ensure accuracy and to prevent errors. Some facilities require the third check to occur at the bedside, after identifying the patient and before administration.

19. **If a multidose vial is being used, label the vial with the date and time opened, and store the vial containing the remaining medication according to facility policy.**

Because the vial is sealed, the medication inside remains sterile and can be used for future injections. Labeling the opened vials with a date and time limits its use after a specific time period.

20. Lock the medication cart before leaving it.

Locking the cart or drawer safeguards the patient's medication supply. Hospital accrediting organizations require medication carts to be locked when not in use.

21. Perform hand hygiene.

Hand hygiene deters the spread of microorganisms.

22. Proceed with administration, based on prescribed route.

See appropriate skill for prescribed route.

EVALUATION   The expected outcome is met when the medication is withdrawn into the syringe in a sterile manner and the proper dose is prepared.

(continued)

Skill · 4 — Removing Medication from a Vial *continued*

DOCUMENTATION

Guidelines

It is not necessary to record the removal of the medication from the vial. Record each medication administered on the CMAR/MAR or record using the required format immediately after it is administered, including date and time of administration. If using a bar-code system, medication administration is automatically recorded when the bar code is scanned. PRN medications require documentation of the reason for administration. Prompt recording avoids the possibility of accidentally repeating the administration of the drug. If the drug was refused or omitted, record this in the appropriate area on the medication record and notify the primary care provider. This verifies the reason medication was omitted and ensures that the primary care provider is aware of the patient's condition. Recording administration of a narcotic may require additional documentation on a narcotic record, stating drug count and other specific information. Record fluid intake if intake and output measurement is required.

UNEXPECTED SITUATIONS AND ASSOCIATED INTERVENTIONS

- *A piece of rubber stopper is noticed floating in medication in syringe:* Discard the syringe, needle, and vial. Obtain a new vial, syringe, and needle and prepare dose as ordered.
- *As needle attached to syringe filled with air is inserted into vial, the plunger is immediately pulled down:* If possible to withdraw medication, continue steps as explained above. If such a vacuum has formed that this is impossible, remove syringe and inject more air into the vial. This is caused by previous withdrawal of medication without the addition of air into the vial.
- *Plunger is contaminated before injecting air into vial:* Discard needle and syringe and start over. If plunger is contaminated after medication is drawn into syringe, it is not necessary to discard and start over. The contaminated plunger will enter the barrel of the syringe when pushing the medication out and will not contaminate the medication.

Skill Variation — Reconstituting Powdered Medication in a Vial

Drugs that are unstable in liquid form are often provided in a dry powder form. The powder must be mixed with the correct amount of appropriate solution to prepare medication for administration. Verify the correct amount and correct solution type for the specific medication prescribed. This information is found on the vial label, package insert, in a drug reference, an on-line pharmacy source, or from the pharmacist. To reconstitute powdered medication:

1. Gather equipment. Check the medication order against the original order in the medical record, according to agency policy.
2. Know the actions, special nursing considerations, safe dose ranges, purpose of administration, and adverse effects of the medications to be administered. Consider the appropriateness of the medication for this patient.

3. Perform hand hygiene.

4. Move the medication cart to the outside of the patient's room or prepare for administration in the medication area.
5. Unlock the medication cart or drawer. Enter pass code and scan employee identification, if required.
6. **Prepare medications for one patient at a time.**
7. Read the CMAR/MAR and select the proper medication and diluent from the patient's medication drawer or unit stock.
8. Compare the labels with the CMAR/MAR. Check expiration dates and perform calculations, check medication calculation with another nurse. Scan the bar code on the package, if required.
9. Remove the metal or plastic cap on the medication vial and diluent vial that protects the self-sealing stoppers.

10. Swab the self-sealing tops with the antimicrobial swab and allow to dry.
11. **Draw up the appropriate amount of diluent into the syringe.**
12. Insert the needle or blunt cannula through the center of the self-sealing stopper on the powdered medication vial.
13. Inject the diluent into the powdered medication vial.
14. Remove the needle or blunt cannula from the vial and replace cap.
15. **Gently agitate the vial to mix the powdered medication and the diluent completely. Do not shake the vial.**
16. **Draw up the prescribed amount of medication while holding the syringe vertically and at eye level.**
17. After the correct dose is withdrawn, remove the needle from the vial and carefully replace the cap over the needle. **If a filter needle has been used to draw up the medication, remove it and attach the appropriate administration device.** Some facilities require changing the needle, if one was used to withdraw the medication, before administering the medication.
18. **Check the amount of medication in the syringe with the medication dose and discard any surplus.**
19. **Recheck the label with the CMAR/MAR.**
20. Lock the medication cart before leaving it.

21. Perform hand hygiene.

22. Proceed with administration, based on prescribed route.

Skill · 5   Mixing Medications From Two Vials in One Syringe

Preparation of medications in one syringe depends on how the medication is supplied. When using a single-dose vial and a multidose vial, air is injected into both vials and the medication in the multidose vial is drawn into the syringe first. This prevents the contents of the multidose vial from being contaminated with the medication in the single-dose vial. The CDC recommends that medications packaged as multiuse vials be assigned to a single patient whenever possible. In addition, it is recommended that the top of the vial be cleaned before each entry, as well as the use of a new sterile needle and syringe (CDC, 2008a; CDC, 2008b).

When considering mixing two medications in one syringe, you must ensure that the two drugs are compatible. Be aware of drug incompatibilities when preparing medications in one syringe. Certain medications, such as diazepam (Valium), are incompatible with other drugs in the same syringe. Other drugs have limited compatibility and should be administered within 15 minutes of preparation. Incompatible drugs may become cloudy or form a precipitate in the syringe. Such medications are discarded and prepared again in separate syringes. Mixing more than two drugs in one syringe is not recommended. If it must be done, contact the pharmacist to determine the compatibility of the three drugs, as well as the compatibility of their pH values and the preservatives that may be present in each drug. A drug-compatibility table should be available to nurses who are preparing medications.

Insulins, with many types available for use, are an example of medications that may be combined together in one syringe for injection. Insulins vary in their onset and duration of action and are classified as rapid acting, short acting, intermediate acting, and long acting. Before administering any insulin, be aware of the onset time, peak, and duration of effects, and ensure that proper food is available. Be aware that some insulins, such as Lantus and Levemir, cannot be mixed with other insulins. Refer to a drug reference for a listing of the different types of insulin and action specific to each type. Insulin dosages are calculated in units. The scale commonly used is U100, which is based on 100 units of insulin contained in 1 mL of solution.

The preparation of two types of insulin in one syringe is used as the example in the following procedure.

EQUIPMENT

- Two vials of medication (insulin in this example)
- Sterile syringe (insulin syringe in this example)
- Antimicrobial swabs
- Computer-generated Medication Administration Record (CMAR) or Medication Administration Record (MAR)

ASSESSMENT

Determine the compatibility of the two medications. Not all insulins can be mixed together. For example, Lantus and Levemir cannot be mixed with other insulins.

Assess the contents of each vial of insulin. It is very important to be familiar with the particular drug's properties to be able to assess the quality of the medication in the vial before withdrawal. Unmodified preparations typically appear as clear substances, so they should be without particles or foreign matter. Modified preparations are typically suspensions, so they do not appear as clear substances. Keep in mind that it is no longer safe to use the terms "clear" and "cloudy" to designate types of insulin preparation. Insulin Glargine (Lantus) is a clear, long-acting insulin (24-hour duration).

Check the expiration date before administering the medication. Assess the appropriateness of the drug for the patient. Review the assessment and laboratory data that may influence drug administration. Check the patient's blood glucose level, if appropriate, before administering the insulin. Verify patient name, dose, route, and time of administration.

NURSING DIAGNOSIS

Determine related factors for the nursing diagnoses based on the patient's current status. Appropriate nursing diagnoses include:

- Risk for Infection
- Deficient Knowledge
- Risk for Injury
- Anxiety

OUTCOME IDENTIFICATION AND PLANNING

The expected outcome to achieve when mixing two different types of medication in one syringe is the accurate withdrawal of the medication into a syringe in a sterile manner and that the proper dose is prepared.

(continued)

Skill · 5   Mixing Medications From Two Vials in One Syringe   *continued*

IMPLEMENTATION

ACTION	RATIONALE
1. Gather equipment. Check medication order against the original order in the medical record, according to facility policy.	This comparison helps to identify errors that may have occurred when orders were transcribed. The primary care provider's order is the legal record of medication orders for each facility.
2. Know the actions, special nursing considerations, safe dose ranges, purpose of administration, and adverse effects of the medications to be administered. Consider the appropriateness of the medication for this patient.	This knowledge aids the nurse in evaluating the therapeutic effect of the medication in relation to the patient's disorder and can also be used to educate the patient about the medication.
3. Perform hand hygiene.	Hand hygiene deters the spread of microorganisms.
4. Move the medication cart to the outside of the patient's room or prepare for administration in the medication area.	Organization facilitates error-free administration and saves time.
5. Unlock the medication cart or drawer. Enter pass code and scan employee identification, if required.	Locking the cart or drawer safeguards each patient's medication supply. Hospital accrediting organizations require medication carts to be locked when not in use. Entering pass code and scanning ID allows only authorized users into the system and identifies user for documentation by the computer.
6. **Prepare medications for one patient at a time.**	This prevents errors in medication administration.
7. Read the CMAR/MAR and select the proper medications from the patient's medication drawer or unit stock.	This is the *first* check of the labels.
8. Compare the labels with the CMAR/MAR. Check expiration dates and perform calculations, if necessary. Scan the bar code on the package, if required.	This is the *second* check of the labels. Verify calculations with another nurse to ensure safety, if necessary.
9. If necessary, remove the cap that protects the rubber stopper on each vial.	The cap protects the rubber top.
10. **If medication is a suspension (e.g., NPH insulin), roll and agitate the vial to mix it well.**	There is controversy regarding how to mix insulins in suspension. Some sources advise rolling the vial; others advise shaking the vial. Consult facility policy. Regardless of the method used, it is essential that the suspension be mixed well to avoid administering an inconsistent dose. Regular insulin, which is clear, does not need to be mixed before withdrawal.
11. Cleanse the rubber tops with antimicrobial swabs.	Antimicrobial swab removes surface contamination. Some sources question whether cleaning with alcohol actually disinfects or instead transfers resident bacteria from the hands to another surface.
12. Remove cap from needle by pulling it straight off. Touch the plunger at the knob only. Draw back an amount of air into the syringe that is equal to the dose of modified insulin to be withdrawn.	Pulling cap off in a straight manner prevents accidental needlestick. Handling the plunger by the knob only ensures sterility of the shaft of the plunger. Before fluid is removed, injection of an equal amount of air is required to prevent the formation of a partial vacuum, because a vial is a sealed container. If not enough air is injected, the negative pressure makes it difficult to withdraw the medication.
13. Hold the modified vial on a flat surface. Pierce the rubber stopper in the center with the needle tip and inject the measured air into the space above the solution (Figure 1). Do not inject air into the solution. Withdraw the needle.	Unmodified insulin should never be contaminated with modified insulin. Placing air in the modified insulin first without allowing the needle to contact the insulin ensures that the second vial-entered (unmodified) insulin is not contaminated by the medication in the other vial. Air bubbled through the solution could result in withdrawal of an inaccurate amount of medication.

ACTION

14. Draw back an amount of air into the syringe that is equal to the dose of unmodified insulin to be withdrawn.

15. Hold the unmodified vial on a flat surface. Pierce the rubber stopper in the center with the needle tip and inject the measured air into the space above the solution (Figure 2). Do not inject air into the solution. Keep the needle in the vial.

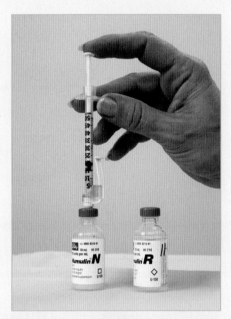

FIGURE 1. Injecting air into modified insulin preparation.

16. Invert vial of unmodified insulin. Hold the vial in one hand and use the other to withdraw the medication. Touch the plunger at the knob only. **Draw up the prescribed amount of medication while holding the syringe at eye level and vertically (Figure 3).** Turn the vial over and then remove needle from vial.

17. Check that there are no air bubbles in the syringe.

18. **Check the amount of medication in the syringe with the medication dose and discard any surplus.**

19. **Recheck the vial label with the CMAR/MAR.**

20. Calculate the endpoint on the syringe for the combined insulin amount by adding the number of units for each dose together.

RATIONALE

Before fluid is removed, injection of an equal amount of air is required to prevent the formation of a partial vacuum, because a vial is a sealed container. If not enough air is injected, the negative pressure makes it difficult to withdraw the medication.

Air bubbled through the solution could result in withdrawal of an inaccurate amount of medication.

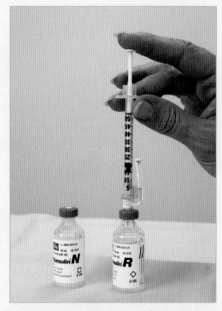

FIGURE 2. Injecting air into the unmodified insulin vial.

Holding the syringe at eye level facilitates accurate reading, and the vertical position makes removal of air bubbles from the syringe easy. First dose is prepared and is not contaminated by insulin that contains modifiers.

The presence of air in the syringe would result in an inaccurate dose of medication.

Careful measurement ensures that correct dose is withdrawn.

This is the *third* check to ensure accuracy and to prevent errors. Some facilities require the third check to occur at the bedside, after identifying the patient and before administration.

Allows for accurate withdrawal of second dose.

(continued)

Skill · 5   Mixing Medications From Two Vials in One Syringe   *continued*

ACTION	RATIONALE
21. Insert the needle into the modified vial and invert it, taking care not to push the plunger and inject medication from the syringe into the vial. Invert vial of modified insulin. Hold the vial in one hand and use the other to withdraw the medication. Touch the plunger at the knob only. **Draw up the prescribed amount of medication while holding the syringe at eye level and vertically (Figure 4). Take care to withdraw only the prescribed amount.** Turn the vial over and then remove needle from vial. Carefully recap the needle. Carefully replace the cap over the needle.	Previous addition of air eliminates need to create positive pressure. Holding the syringe at eye level facilitates accurate reading. Capping the needle prevents contamination and protects the nurse against accidental needlesticks. A one-handed recap method may be used as long as care is taken to ensure that the needle remains sterile.

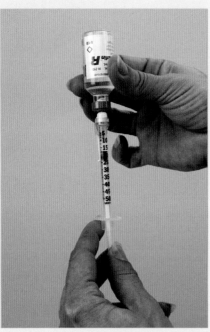

FIGURE 3. Withdrawing the prescribed amount of unmodified insulin.

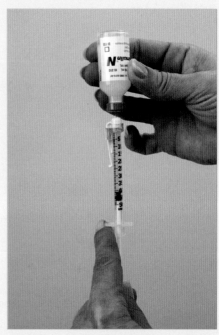

FIGURE 4. Withdrawing modified insulin.

22. **Check the amount of medication in the syringe with the medication dose.**	Careful measurement ensures that correct dose is withdrawn.
23. **Recheck the vial label with the CMAR/MAR.**	This is the *third* check to ensure accuracy and to prevent errors. Some facilities require the third check to occur at the bedside, after identifying the patient and before administration.
24. **Label the vials with the date and time opened, and store the vials containing the remaining medication according to facility policy.**	Because the vial is sealed, the medication inside remains sterile and can be used for future injections. Labeling the opened vials with a date and time limits its use after a specific time period. The CDC recommends that medications packaged as multiuse vials be assigned to a single patient whenever possible (CDC, 2008a; CDC, 2008b).
25. Lock medication cart before leaving it.	Locking the cart or drawer safeguards the patient's medication supply. Hospital accrediting organizations require medication carts to be locked when not in use.
26. Perform hand hygiene.	Hand hygiene deters the spread of microorganisms.
27. Proceed with administration, based on prescribed route.	See appropriate skill for prescribed route.

EVALUATION

The expected outcome is met when the medication is withdrawn into a syringe in a sterile manner, and the proper dose is prepared.

DOCUMENTATION

Guidelines

It is not necessary to record the removal of the medication from the vials. Record each medication administered on the CMAR/MAR or record using the required format immediately after it is administered, including date and time of administration. If using a bar-code system, medication administration is automatically recorded when the bar code is scanned. PRN medications require documentation of the reason for administration. Prompt recording avoids the possibility of accidentally repeating the administration of the drug. If the drug was refused or omitted, record this in the appropriate area on the medication record and notify the primary care provider. This verifies the reason medication was omitted and ensures that the primary care provider is aware of the patient's condition. Recording administration of a narcotic may require additional documentation on a narcotic record, stating drug count and other specific information.

UNEXPECTED SITUATIONS AND ASSOCIATED INTERVENTIONS

- *You contaminate plunger before injecting air into insulin vial:* Discard needle and syringe and start over. If plunger is contaminated after medication is drawn into the syringe, it is not necessary to discard and start over. The contaminated plunger will enter the barrel of the syringe when pushing the medication out and will not contaminate the medication.
- *You allow modified insulin to come in contact with the needle before entering the unmodified insulin vial:* Discard needle and syringe and start over.
- *You notice that the combined amount is not the ordered amount (e.g., you have less or more units in combined syringe than ordered):* Discard syringe and start over. There is no way to know for sure which dosage is wrong or which medication should be expelled.
- *You inject medication from first vial (in syringe) into second vial:* Discard vial and syringe and start over.

SPECIAL CONSIDERATIONS

General Considerations

- A patient with diabetes who is visually impaired may find it helpful to use a magnifying apparatus that fits around the syringe.
- Before attempting to explain or demonstrate devices that help low-vision diabetic patients to prepare their medication, attempt to use the device yourself under similar circumstances. To detect any difficulties the patient may experience, practice using the aid with your eyes closed or in a poorly lit room.

Infant and Child Considerations

School-age children are generally able to prepare and administer their own injections, such as insulin, with supervision (Kyle, 2008). Parents/significant others and the child should be involved in teaching.

Skill · 6   Administering an Intradermal Injection

Intradermal injections are administered into the dermis, just below the epidermis. The intradermal route has the longest absorption time of all parenteral routes. For this reason, intradermal injections are used for sensitivity tests, such as tuberculin and allergy tests, and local anesthesia. The advantage of the intradermal route for these tests is that the body's reaction to substances is easily visible, and degrees of reaction are discernible by comparative study.

Sites commonly used are the inner surface of the forearm and the upper back, under the scapula. Equipment used for an intradermal injection includes a tuberculin syringe calibrated in tenths and hundredths of a milliliter and a ¼- to ½-inch, 26- or 27-gauge needle. The dosage given intradermally is small, usually less than 0.5 mL. The angle of administration for an intradermal injection is 5 to 15 degrees (see Figure 5-1 in the chapter opener).

(continued)

Skill · 6 Administering an Intradermal Injection *continued*

EQUIPMENT

- Prescribed medication
- Sterile syringe, usually a tuberculin syringe calibrated in tenths and hundredths, and needle, ¼- to ½-inch, 26- or 27-gauge
- Antimicrobial swab
- Disposable gloves
- Small gauze square
- Computer-generated Medication Administration Record (CMAR) or Medication Administration Record (MAR)
- PPE, as indicated

ASSESSMENT

Assess the patient for any allergies. Check expiration date before administering medication. Assess the appropriateness of the drug for the patient. Review assessment and laboratory data that may influence drug administration. Assess the site on the patient where the injection is to be given. Avoid areas of broken or open skin. Avoid areas that are highly pigmented, and those that have lesions, bruises, or scars and are hairy. Assess the patient's knowledge of the medication. This may provide an opportune time for patient education. Verify the patient's name, dose, route, and time of administration.

NURSING DIAGNOSIS

Determine related factors for the nursing diagnoses based on the patient's current status. Appropriate nursing diagnoses may include:

- Deficient Knowledge
- Risk for Infection
- Anxiety
- Risk for Allergy Response
- Risk for Injury

OUTCOME IDENTIFICATION AND PLANNING

The expected outcome to achieve when administering an intradermal injection is the appearance of a wheal at the site of injection. Other outcomes that may be appropriate include the following: the patient refrains from rubbing the site; the patient's anxiety is decreased; the patient does not experience adverse effects; and the patient understands and complies with the medication regimen.

IMPLEMENTATION

ACTION	RATIONALE
1. Gather equipment. Check each medication order against the original order in the medical record according to facility policy. Clarify any inconsistencies. Check the patient's chart for allergies.	This comparison helps to identify errors that may have occurred when orders were transcribed. The primary care provider's order is the legal record of medication orders for each facility.
2. Know the actions, special nursing considerations, safe dose ranges, purpose of administration, and adverse effects of the medications to be administered. Consider the appropriateness of the medication for this patient.	This knowledge aids the nurse in evaluating the therapeutic effect of the medication in relation to the patient's disorder and can also be used to educate the patient about the medication.
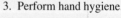 3. Perform hand hygiene.	Hand hygiene prevents the spread of microorganisms.
4. Move the medication cart to the outside of the patient's room or prepare for administration in the medication area.	Organization facilitates error-free administration and saves time.
5. Unlock the medication cart or drawer. Enter pass code and scan employee identification, if required.	Locking the cart or drawer safeguards each patient's medication supply. Hospital accrediting organizations require medication carts to be locked when not in use. Entering pass code and scanning ID allows only authorized users into the system and identifies user for documentation by the computer.
6. **Prepare medications for one patient at a time.**	This prevents errors in medication administration.
7. Read the CMAR/MAR and select the proper medication from the patient's medication drawer or unit stock.	This is the *first* check of the label.

ACTION	RATIONALE

8. Compare the label with the CMAR/MAR. Check expiration dates and perform calculations, if necessary. Scan the bar code on the package, if required.

This is the *second* check of the label. Verify calculations with another nurse to ensure safety.

9. If necessary, withdraw medication from an ampule or vial as described in Skills 5-3 and 5-4.

10. **When all medications for one patient have been prepared, recheck the label with the CMAR/MAR before taking the medications to the patient.**

This is a *third* check to ensure accuracy and to prevent errors. Some facilities require the third check to occur at the bedside, after identifying the patient and before administration.

11. Lock the medication cart before leaving it.

Locking the cart or drawer safeguards the patient's medication supply. Hospital accrediting organizations require medication carts to be locked when not in use.

12. Transport medications to the patient's bedside carefully, and keep the medications in sight at all times.

Careful handling and close observation prevent accidental or deliberate disarrangement of medications.

13. **Ensure that the patient receives the medications at the correct time.**

Check agency policy, which may allow for administration within a period of 30 minutes before or 30 minutes after the designated time.

14. Perform hand hygiene and put on PPE, if indicated.

Hand hygiene and PPE prevent the spread of microorganisms. PPE is required based on transmission precautions.

15. Identify the patient. Usually, the patient should be identified using two methods. Compare information with the CMAR/MAR.

Identifying the patient ensures the right patient receives the medications and helps prevent errors.

   a. Check the name and identification number on the patient's identification band.

This is the most reliable method. Replace the identification band if it is missing or inaccurate in any way.

   b. Ask the patient to state his or her name and birth date, based on facility policy.

This requires a response from the patient, but illness and strange surroundings often cause patients to be confused.

   c. If the patient cannot identify him- or herself, verify the patient's identification with a staff member who knows the patient for the second source.

This is another way to double-check identity. Do not use the name on the door or over the bed, because these signs may be inaccurate.

16. Close the door to the room or pull the bedside curtain.

This provides patient privacy.

17. Complete necessary assessments before administering medications. Check allergy bracelet or ask the patient about allergies. Explain the purpose and action of the medication to the patient.

Assessment is a prerequisite to administration of medications. Explanation provides rationale, increases knowledge, and reduces anxiety.

18. Scan the patient's bar code on the identification band, if required.

Provides an additional check to ensure that the medication is given to the right patient.

19. Put on clean gloves.

Gloves help prevent exposure to contaminants.

20. Select an appropriate administration site. Assist the patient to the appropriate position for the site chosen. Drape as needed to expose only area of site to be used.

Appropriate site prevents injury and allows for accurate reading of the test site at the appropriate time. Draping provides privacy and warmth.

21. Cleanse the site with an antimicrobial swab while wiping with a firm, circular motion and moving outward from the injection site. Allow the skin to dry.

Pathogens on the skin can be forced into the tissues by the needle. Moving from the center outward prevents contamination of the site. Allowing skin to dry prevents introducing alcohol into the tissue, which can be irritating and uncomfortable.

22. Remove the needle cap with the nondominant hand by pulling it straight off.

This technique lessens the risk of an accidental needlestick.

23. Use the nondominant hand to spread the skin taut over the injection site (Figure 1).

Taut skin provides an easy entrance into intradermal tissue.

(continued)

Skill · 6   **Administering an Intradermal Injection**   *continued*

ACTION

24. Hold the syringe in the dominant hand, between the thumb and forefinger with the bevel of the needle up.

25. Hold the syringe at a 5- to 15-degree angle from the site. **Place the needle almost flat against the patient's skin (Figure 2), bevel side up, and insert the needle into the skin. Insert the needle only about ⅛ inch with entire bevel under the skin.**

RATIONALE

Using the dominant hand allows for easy, appropriate handling of the syringe. Having the bevel up allows for smooth piercing of the skin and introduction of medication into the dermis.

The dermis is entered when the needle is held as nearly parallel to the skin as possible and is inserted about ⅛ inch.

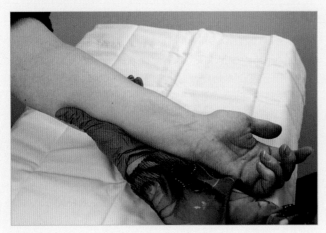

FIGURE 1. Spreading the skin taut over the injection site.

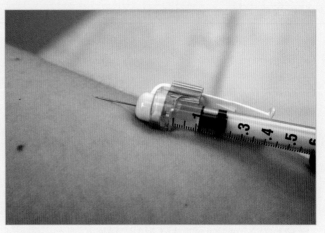

FIGURE 2. Inserting the needle almost level with the skin.

26. Once the needle is in place, steady the lower end of the syringe. Slide your dominant hand to the end of the plunger.

27. Slowly inject the agent while watching for a small wheal or blister to appear (Figure 3).

Prevents injury and inadvertent advancement or withdrawal of needle.

The appearance of a wheal indicates the medication is in the dermis.

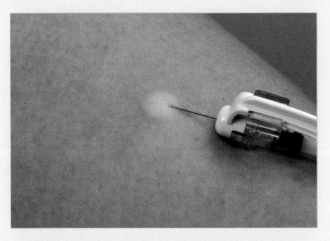

FIGURE 3. Observing for wheal while injecting medication.

28. Withdraw the needle quickly at the same angle that it was inserted. Do not recap the used needle. Engage the safety shield or needle guard.

29. **Do not massage the area after removing needle. Tell patient not to rub or scratch the site. If necessary, gently blot the site with a dry gauze square. Do not apply pressure or rub the site.**

Withdrawing the needle quickly and at the angle at which it entered the skin minimizes tissue damage and discomfort for the patient. Safety shield or needle guard prevents accidental needlestick injury.

Massaging the area where an intradermal injection is given may spread the medication to underlying subcutaneous tissue.

ACTION	RATIONALE
30. Assist the patient to a position of comfort.	This provides for the well-being of the patient.
31. Discard the needle and syringe in the appropriate receptacle.	Proper disposal of the needle prevents injury.
32. Remove gloves and additional PPE, if used. Perform hand hygiene.	Removing PPE properly reduces the risk for infection transmission and contamination of other items. Hand hygiene prevents the spread of microorganisms.
33. Document the administration of the medication immediately after administration. See Documentation section below.	Timely documentation helps to ensure patient safety.
34. Evaluate the patient's response to medication within appropriate time frame.	The patient needs to be evaluated for therapeutic and adverse effects from the medication.
35. Observe the area for signs of a reaction at determined intervals after administration. Inform the patient of the need for inspection.	With many intradermal injections, you need to look for a localized reaction in the area of the injection at the appropriate interval(s) determined by the type of medication and purpose. Explaining this to the patient increases compliance.

EVALUATION

The expected outcomes are met when you note a wheal at site of injection; the patient refrains from rubbing the site; the patient's anxiety is decreased; the patient did not experience adverse effects; and the patient verbalizes an understanding of, and complies with, the medication regimen.

DOCUMENTATION

Guidelines

Record each medication administered on the CMAR/MAR or record using the required format, including date, time, and the site of administration, immediately after administration. Some facilities recommend circling the injection site with ink. Circling the injection site easily identifies the site of the intradermal injection and allows for future careful observation of the exact area. If using a bar-code system, medication administration is automatically recorded when the bar code is scanned. PRN medications require documentation of the reason for administration. Prompt recording avoids the possibility of accidentally repeating the administration of the drug. If the drug was refused or omitted, record this in the appropriate area on the medication record and notify the primary care provider. This verifies the reason medication was omitted and ensures that the primary care provider is aware of the patient's condition.

UNEXPECTED SITUATIONS AND ASSOCIATED INTERVENTIONS

- *You do not note wheal or blister at site of injection:* Medication has been injected subcutaneously. Document according to facility policy and inform the primary care provider. You may need to obtain an order to repeat the procedure.
- *Medication leaks out of injection site before needle is withdrawn:* Needle was inserted less than ⅛ inch. Document according to facility policy and inform the primary care provider. You may need to obtain an order to repeat the procedure.
- *You stick yourself with the needle before injection:* Discard needle and syringe appropriately. Follow facility policy regarding needlestick injury. Prepare new syringe with medication and administer to patient. Complete appropriate paperwork and follow facility's policy regarding accidental needlestick injuries.
- *You stick yourself with needle after injection:* Discard needle and syringe appropriately. Follow facility policy regarding needlestick injury. Complete appropriate paperwork and follow facility's policy regarding accidental needlesticks.

SPECIAL CONSIDERATIONS

- Ongoing assessment is an important part of nursing care for both evaluation of patient response to administered medications and early detection of adverse effects. If an adverse effect is suspected, withhold further medication doses and notify the patient's primary healthcare provider. Additional intervention is based on type of reaction and patient assessment.
- Aspiration, pulling back on the plunger after insertion and before administration, is not recommended for an intradermal injection. The dermis does not contain large blood vessels.
- Some agencies recommend administering intradermal injections with the bevel down instead of the bevel up. Check facility policy.

Skill · 7   Administering a Subcutaneous Injection

Subcutaneous injections are administered into the adipose tissue layer just below the epidermis and dermis. This tissue has few blood vessels, so drugs administered here have a slow, sustained rate of absorption into the capillaries.

It is important to choose the right equipment to ensure depositing the medication into the intended tissue layer and not the underlying muscle. Equipment used for a subcutaneous injection includes a syringe of appropriate volume for the amount of drug being administered. An insulin pen may be used for subcutaneous injection of insulin (see the accompanying Skill Variation for technique). A 25- to 30-gauge, ⅜- to 1-inch needle can be used; ⅜- and ⅝-inch sized needles are most commonly used. Some medications are packaged in prefilled cartridges with a needle attached. Confirm that the provided needle is appropriate for the patient before use. If not, the medication will have to be transferred to another syringe and the appropriate needle attached.

Review the specifics of the particular medication before administrating it to the patient. Various sites may be used for subcutaneous injections, including the outer aspect of the upper arm, the abdomen (from below the costal margin to the iliac crests), the anterior aspects of the thigh, the upper back, and the upper ventral gluteal area. Figure 1 displays the sites on the body where subcutaneous injections can be given. Absorption rates are different from the different sites. Injections in the abdomen are absorbed most rapidly, absorbed somewhat slower from the arms, even slower from the thighs, and slowest from the upper ventral gluteal areas (American Diabetes Association, 2004; Caffrey, 2003).

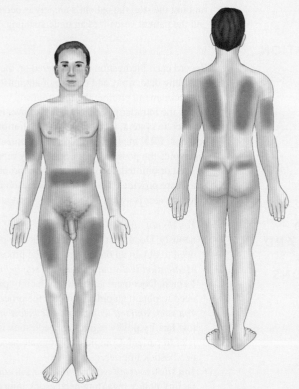

FIGURE 1. Sites on the body where subcutaneous injections can be given.

Subcutaneous injections are administered at a 45- to 90-degree angle. Choose the angle of needle insertion based on the amount of subcutaneous tissue present and the length of the needle. Choose the needle length based on the amount of subcutaneous tissue present, based on the patient's body weight and build (Annersten & Willman, 2005). Generally, insert the shorter, ⅜-inch needle at a 90-degree angle and the longer, ⅝-inch needle at a 45-degree angle. Figure 5-1 in the chapter opener shows the angles of insertion for subcutaneous injections.

Recommendations differ regarding pinching or bunching of a skin fold for administration. Pinching is advised for thinner patients and when a longer needle is used, to lift the adipose tissue away from underlying muscle and tissue. If pinching is used, once the needle is inserted, release the skin to avoid injecting into compressed tissue (Rushing, 2004).

Aspiration, or pulling back on the plunger to check that a blood vessel has been entered, is not necessary and has not proved to be a reliable indicator of needle placement. The likelihood of injecting into a blood vessel is small (Rushing, 2004; Stephens, 2003). The American Diabetes Association (2004) has stated that routine aspiration is not necessary when injecting insulin. Aspiration is definitely contraindicated with administration of heparin because this action can result in hematoma formation.

Usually, no more than 1 mL of solution is given subcutaneously. Giving larger amounts adds to the patient's discomfort and may predispose to poor absorption.

EQUIPMENT

- Prescribed medication
- Sterile syringe and needle. Needle size depends on the medication administered and patient body type (see previous discussion).
- Antimicrobial swab
- Disposable gloves
- Small gauze square
- Computer-generated Medication Administration Record (CMAR) or Medication Administration Record (MAR)
- PPE, as indicated

ASSESSMENT

Assess the patient for any allergies. Check expiration date before administering medication. Assess the appropriateness of the drug for the patient. Verify patient name, dose, route, and time of administration. Review assessment and laboratory data that may influence drug administration. Assess the site on the patient where the injection is to be given. Avoid sites that are bruised, tender, hard, swollen, inflamed, or scarred. These conditions could affect absorption or cause discomfort and injury (Hunter, 2008). Assess the patient's knowledge of the medication. If the patient has deficient knowledge about the medication, this may be the appropriate time to begin education about it. If the medication may affect the patient's vital signs, assess them before administration. If the medication is for pain relief, assess the patient's pain before and after administration.

NURSING DIAGNOSIS

Determine related factors for the nursing diagnoses based on the patient's current status. Appropriate nursing diagnoses may include:
- Deficient Knowledge
- Risk for Infection
- Risk for Allergy Response
- Acute Pain
- Risk for Injury
- Anxiety

OUTCOME IDENTIFICATION AND PLANNING

The expected outcome is that the patient receives medication via the subcutaneous route. Other outcomes that may be appropriate include the following: the patient's anxiety is decreased; the patient does not experience adverse effects; and the patient understands and complies with the medication regimen.

IMPLEMENTATION

ACTION	RATIONALE
1. Gather equipment. Check each medication order against the original order in the medical record, according to facility policy. Clarify any inconsistencies. Check the patient's chart for allergies.	This comparison helps to identify errors that may have occurred when orders were transcribed. The primary care provider's order is the legal record of medication orders for each facility.
2. Know the actions, special nursing considerations, safe dose ranges, purpose of administration, and adverse effects of the medications to be administered. Consider the appropriateness of the medication for this patient.	This knowledge aids the nurse in evaluating the therapeutic effect of the medication in relation to the patient's disorder and can also be used to educate the patient about the medication.
3. Perform hand hygiene.	Hand hygiene prevents the spread of microorganisms.

(continued)

Skill · 7   Administering a Subcutaneous Injection   *continued*

ACTION	RATIONALE
4. Move the medication cart to the outside of the patient's room or prepare for administration in the medication area.	Organization facilitates error-free administration and saves time.
5. Unlock the medication cart or drawer. Enter pass code and scan employee identification, if required.	Locking the cart or drawer safeguards each patient's medication supply. Hospital accrediting organizations require medication carts to be locked when not in use. Entering pass code and scanning ID allows only authorized users into the system and identifies user for documentation by the computer.
6. **Prepare medications for one patient at a time.**	This prevents errors in medication administration.
7. Read the CMAR/MAR and select the proper medication from the patient's medication drawer or unit stock.	This is the *first* check of the label.
8. Compare the label with the CMAR/MAR. Check expiration dates and perform calculations, if necessary. Scan the bar code on the package, if required.	This is the *second* check of the label. Verify calculations with another nurse to ensure safety, if necessary.
9. If necessary, withdraw medication from an ampule or vial as described in Skills 5-3 and 5-4.	
10. **When all medications for one patient have been prepared, recheck the label with the MAR before taking medications to the patient.**	This is a *third* check to ensure accuracy and to prevent errors. Some facilities require the third check to occur at the bedside, after identifying the patient and before administration.
11. Lock the medication cart before leaving it.	Locking the cart or drawer safeguards the patient's medication supply. Hospital accrediting organizations require medication carts to be locked when not in use.
12. Transport medications to the patient's bedside carefully, and keep the medications in sight at all times.	Careful handling and close observation prevent accidental or deliberate disarrangement of medications.
13. **Ensure that the patient receives the medications at the correct time.**	Check agency policy, which may allow for administration within a period of 30 minutes before or 30 minutes after the designated time.
14. Perform hand hygiene and put on PPE, if indicated.	Hand hygiene and PPE prevent the spread of microorganisms. PPE is required based on transmission precautions.
15. Identify the patient. Usually, the patient should be identified using two methods. Compare information with the CMAR/MAR.	Identifying the patient ensures the right patient receives the medications and helps prevent errors.
a. Check the name and identification number on the patient's identification band.	This is the most reliable method. Replace the identification band if it is missing or inaccurate in any way.
b. Ask the patient to state his or her name and birth date, based on facility policy.	This requires a response from the patient, but illness and strange surroundings often cause patients to be confused.
c. If the patient cannot identify him- or herself, verify the patient's identification with a staff member who knows the patient for the second source.	This is another way to double-check identity. Do not use the name on the door or over the bed, because these signs may be inaccurate.
16. Close the door to the room or pull the bedside curtain.	This provides patient privacy.
17. Complete necessary assessments before administering medications. Check the patient's allergy bracelet or ask the patient about allergies. Explain the purpose and action of the medication to the patient.	Assessment is a prerequisite to administration of medications. Explanation provides rationale, increases knowledge, and reduces anxiety.
18. Scan the patient's bar code on the identification band, if required.	Scanning provides an additional check to ensure that the medication is given to the right patient.
19. Put on clean gloves.	Gloves help prevent exposure to contaminants.
20. Select an appropriate administration site.	Appropriate site prevents injury and allows for accurate reading of the test site at the appropriate time.

ACTION

21. Assist the patient to the appropriate position for the site chosen. Drape, as needed, to expose only area of site to be used.

22. Identify the appropriate landmarks for the site chosen.

23. Cleanse the area around the injection site with an antimicrobial swab. Use a firm, circular motion while moving outward from the injection site (Figure 2). Allow area to dry.

24. Remove the needle cap with the nondominant hand, pulling it straight off.

25. Grasp and bunch the area surrounding the injection site or spread the skin taut at the site (Figure 3).

RATIONALE

Appropriate site prevents injury. Draping helps maintain the patient's privacy.

Good visualization is necessary to establish the correct location of the site and to avoid damage to tissues.

Pathogens on the skin can be forced into the tissues by the needle. Moving from the center outward prevents contamination of the site. Allowing skin to dry prevents introducing alcohol into the tissue, which can be irritating and uncomfortable.

The cap protects the needle from contact with microorganisms. This technique lessens the risk of an accidental needlestick.

Decision to create a skin fold is based on the nurse's assessment of the patient and needle length used. Pinching is advised for thinner patients and when a longer needle is used, to lift the adipose tissue away from underlying muscle and tissue. If pinching is used, once the needle is inserted, release the skin to avoid injecting into compressed tissue. If skin is pulled taut, it provides easy, less painful entry into the subcutaneous tissue.

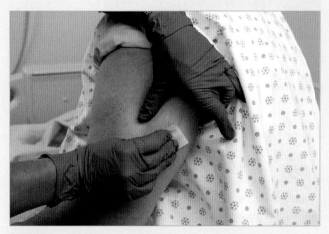

FIGURE 2. Cleaning injection site.

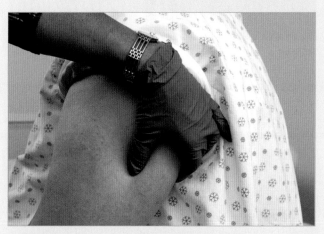

FIGURE 3. Bunching tissue around injection site.

26. **Hold the syringe in the dominant hand between the thumb and forefinger. Inject the needle quickly at a 45- to 90-degree angle (Figure 4).**

27. After the needle is in place, release the tissue. If you have a large skin fold pinched up, ensure that the needle stays in place as the skin is released. Immediately move your nondominant hand to steady the lower end of the syringe. Slide your dominant hand to the end of the plunger. Avoid moving the syringe.

28. Inject the medication slowly (at a rate of 10 sec/mL).

29. Withdraw the needle quickly at the same angle at which it was inserted, while supporting the surrounding tissue with your nondominant hand.

Inserting the needle quickly causes less pain to the patient. Subcutaneous tissue is abundant in well-nourished, well-hydrated people and spare in emaciated, dehydrated, or very thin persons. For a person with little subcutaneous tissue, it is best to insert the needle at a 45-degree angle.

Injecting the solution into compressed tissues results in pressure against nerve fibers and creates discomfort. If there is a large skin fold, the skin may retract away from the needle. The nondominant hand secures the syringe. Moving the syringe could cause damage to the tissues and inadvertent administration into incorrect area.

Rapid injection of the solution creates pressure in the tissues, resulting in discomfort.

Slow withdrawal of the needle pulls the tissues and causes discomfort. Applying counter traction around the injection site helps to prevent pulling on the tissue as the needle is withdrawn. Removing the needle at the same angle at which it was inserted minimizes tissue damage and discomfort for the patient.

(continued)

Skill · 7 Administering a Subcutaneous Injection *continued*

ACTION

RATIONALE

30. Using a gauze square, apply gentle pressure to the site after the needle is withdrawn (Figure 5). Do not massage the site.

Massaging the site is not necessary and can damage underlying tissue and increase the absorption of the medication. Massaging after heparin administration can contribute to hematoma formation. Massaging after an insulin injection may contribute to unpredictable absorption of the medication.

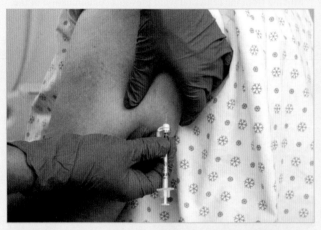

FIGURE 4. Inserting needle.

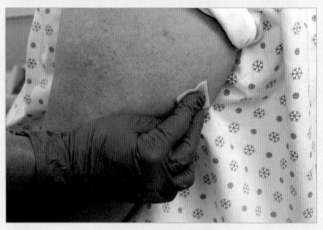

FIGURE 5. Applying pressure to the injection site.

31. Do not recap the used needle. Engage the safety shield or needle guard. Discard the needle and syringe in the appropriate receptacle.

Safety shield or needle guard prevents accidental needlestick. Proper disposal of the needle prevents injury.

32. Assist the patient to a position of comfort.

This provides for the well-being of the patient.

33. Remove gloves and additional PPE, if used. Perform hand hygiene.

Removing PPE properly reduces the risk for infection transmission and contamination of other items. Hand hygiene prevents the spread of microorganisms.

34. Document the administration of the medication immediately after administration. See Documentation section below.

Timely documentation helps to ensure patient safety.

35. Evaluate the patient's response to the medication within an appropriate time frame for the particular medication.

The patient needs to be evaluated for therapeutic and adverse effects from the medication.

EVALUATION

The expected outcomes are met when the patient receives the medication via the subcutaneous route; the patient's anxiety is decreased; the patient does not experience adverse effects; and the patient understands and complies with the medication regimen.

DOCUMENTATION

Guidelines

Record each medication given on the CMAR/MAR or record using the required format, including date, dose, time, and the site of administration, immediately after administration. If using a bar-code system, medication administration is automatically recorded when the bar code is scanned. PRN medications require documentation of the reason for administration. Prompt recording avoids the possibility of accidentally repeating the administration of the drug. If the drug was refused or omitted, record this in the appropriate area on the medication record and notify the primary care provider. This verifies the reason medication was omitted and ensures that the primary care provider is aware of the patient's condition.

UNEXPECTED SITUATIONS AND ASSOCIATED INTERVENTIONS

- *When skin fold is released, needle pulls out of skin:* Engage safety shield or needle guard. Appropriately discard needle. Attach new needle to syringe and administer injection.
- *Patient refuses to let you administer medication in a different location:* Explain the rationale behind rotating injection sites. Discuss other available injection sites with the patient. If the patient will still not allow injection in another area, administer medication to patient, document patient's refusal and discussion, and notify primary care provider.
- *You stick yourself with needle before injection:* Discard needle and syringe appropriately. Follow facility policy regarding needlestick injury. Prepare new syringe with medication and administer to patient. Complete appropriate paperwork and follow facility's policy regarding accidental needlestick injuries.
- *You stick yourself with needle after injection:* Discard needle and syringe appropriately. Complete appropriate paperwork and follow facility's policy regarding accidental needlestick injuries.
- *During injection, patient pulls away from needle before medication is delivered fully:* Remove and appropriately discard needle. Attach a new needle to syringe and administer remaining medication at a different site. Document events and interventions according to facility policy.

SPECIAL CONSIDERATIONS

General Considerations

- Ongoing assessment is an important part of nursing care for both evaluation of patient response to administered medications and early detection of adverse effects. If an adverse effect is suspected, withhold further medication doses and notify the patient's primary healthcare provider. Additional intervention is based on type of reaction and patient assessment.
- Heparin is also administered subcutaneously. The abdomen is the most commonly used site. Avoid the area 2 inches around the umbilicus and the belt line. The manufacturer's (Sanofi Aventis, 2007) directions for subcutaneous administration of low–molecular-weight heparin preparations, such as enoxaparin (Lovenox), include specific instructions regarding administration site and technique. Administer enoxaparin in an area on the abdomen between the left or right anterolateral and left or right posterolateral abdominal wall (Figure 6). To administer the medication, pinch the tissue gently and insert the needle at a 90-degree angle. In addition, enoxaparin is packaged in a prefilled syringe with an air bubble. Do not expel the air bubble before administration.

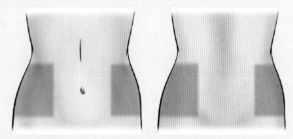

Anterior view   Posterior view

FIGURE 6. Sites for administration of enoxaparin.

Infant and Child Considerations

- Do not tell a child that an injection will not hurt. Describe the feel of the injection as a pinch or a sting. A child who believes you have been dishonest with him or her is less likely to cooperate with future procedures.

Older Adult Considerations

- Many elderly patients have less adipose tissue. Adjust the angle of the needle and angle of insertion accordingly. You do not want to inadvertently give a subcutaneous medication intramuscularly.

Home Care Considerations

- Reuse of syringes in the home setting is not recommended.
- Changes and improvements to insulin syringes to make injections painless have resulted in thinner, shorter, sharper, and better lubricated needles. As a result, after one injection the tip of the fine needles can bend and form a hook that can tear tissue if reused. In addition, these fine needles can break and leave fragments in the skin and tissue if reused. Reuse results in more painful injections related to a reduction in needle lubricant and tip damage (Caffrey, 2003).
- Encourage patients to consult the policies of their local government regarding contaminated and sharps waste disposal. It is important to dispose of needles and syringes in a hard, plastic container. Liquid detergent or liquid fabric softener containers are good choices. Never use glass containers.

(continued)

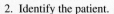

Skill · 7   **Administering a Subcutaneous Injection**   *continued*

Skill Variation   **Using an Insulin Pen to Administer Insulin via the Subcutaneous Route**

1. Perform hand hygiene and put on PPE, as indicated.

2. Identify the patient.

3. Explain procedure to patient.
4. Remove the pen cap.
5. Insert an insulin cartridge into the pen, following the manufacturer's directions.
6. Clean the tip of the reservoir with alcohol.
7. Invert the pen 20 times to mix if using an insulin suspension.
8. Remove the protective tab from the needle.
9. Screw the needle onto the reservoir.
10. Remove the outer and inner needle caps.
11. Hold the pen upright and tap to force any air bubbles to the top.
12. Dial the dose selector to 2 units to perform an "air shot" to get rid of bubbles.
13. Hold the pen upright and press the plunger firmly. Watch for a drop of insulin at the needle tip.
14. Check the drug reservoir to make sure sufficient insulin is available for the dose.
15. Check that the dose selector is at "0," then dial the units of insulin for the dose.
16. Put on gloves.
17. Clean the injection site and administer the subcutaneous injection, holding the pen like a dart. Push the button on the pen all the way in (Figure A).

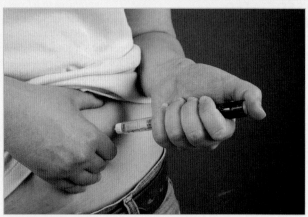
FIGURE A. Patient using insulin pen.

18. Keep the button depressed and count to 6 before removing from the skin.
19. Remove the needle from the pen and dispose in a sharps container.
20. Remove gloves and additional PPE, if used.

21. Perform hand hygiene.

22. Document administration on the CMAR/MAR, including the injection site.

(Adapted from Moshang, J. (2005). Making a point about insulin pens. *Nursing*, 35(2), 46–47.)

Skill · 8   **Administering an Intramuscular Injection**

Intramuscular injections deliver medication through the skin and subcutaneous tissues into certain muscles. Muscles have a larger and a greater number of blood vessels than subcutaneous tissue, allowing faster onset of action than with subcutaneous injections. An intramuscular injection is chosen when a reasonably rapid systemic uptake of the drug is needed by the body and when a relatively prolonged action is required (Hunter & Clark, 2008). Some medications administered intramuscularly are formulated to have a longer duration of effect. The deposit of medication creates a depot at the site of injection, designed to deliver slow, sustained release over hours, days, or weeks.

To administer an intramuscular injection correctly and effectively, choose the right equipment, select the appropriate location, use the correct technique, and deliver the correct dose. Inject the medication into the denser part of the muscle fascia below the subcutaneous tissues. This is ideal because skeletal muscles have fewer pain-sensing nerves than subcutaneous tissue and can absorb larger volumes of solution because of the rapid uptake of the drug into the bloodstream via the muscle fibers (Hunter, 2008).

It is important to choose the right needle length for a particular intramuscular injection. Needle length should be based on the site for injection and the patient's age. See Table 5-1 for intramuscular needle length recommendations. Patients who are obese may require a longer needle, and emaciated patients may require a shorter needle. Appropriate gauge is determined by the medication being administered. Generally, biologic agents and medications in aqueous solutions should be administered with a 20- to 25-gauge needle. Medications in oil-based solutions should be administered with an 18- to 25-gauge needle. Many medications come in prefilled syringe units. If a needle is provided on the prefilled unit, ensure that the needle on the unit is the appropriate length for the patient and situation.

To avoid complications, be able to identify anatomic landmarks and site boundaries. See Figure 1 for a depiction of anatomic landmarks and site boundaries for potential intramuscular injection sites.

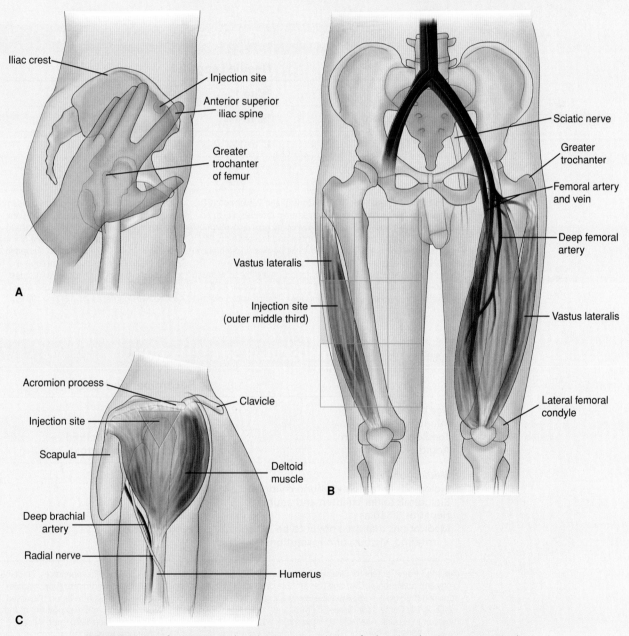

FIGURE 1. Sites for intramuscular injections. Descriptions for locating the sites are given in the text. (**A**) The ventrogluteal site is located by placing the palm on the greater trochanter and the index finger toward the anterosuperior iliac spine. (**B**) The vastus lateralis site is identified by dividing the thigh into thirds, horizontally and vertically. (**C**) The deltoid muscle site is located by palpating the lower edge of the acromion process.

(continued)

Skill · 8   **Administering an Intramuscular Injection**   *continued*

Consider the age of the patient, medication type, and medication volume when selecting a site for intramuscular injection. See Table 5-2 for information related to intramuscular site selection. Rotate the sites used to administer intramuscular medications when therapy requires repeated injections. Whatever pattern of rotating sites is used, a description of it should appear in the patient's plan of nursing care. Depending on the site selected, it may be necessary to reposition the patient (see Table 5-3).

   Use accurate, careful technique when administering intramuscular injections. If care is not taken, possible complications include abscesses; cellulites; injury to blood vessels, bones, and nerves; lingering pain; tissue necrosis; and periostitis (inflammation of the membrane covering a bone). Administer the intramuscular injection so that the needle is perpendicular to the patient's body. This

TABLE · 8-1   INTRAMUSCULAR INJECTION NEEDLE LENGTH

Site/Age	Needle Length
Vastus lateralis	⅝″ to 1″
Deltoid (children)	⅝″ to 1¼″
Deltoid (adults)	1″ to 1½″
Ventrogluteal (adults)	1½″

(Adapted from Centers for Disease Control and Prevention (CDC). (2009). *The pink book*: Appendices. Epidemiology and prevention of vaccine preventable diseases. (11th ed.). Appendix D. Vaccine administration. Vaccine administration guidelines. Available www.cdc.gov/vaccines/pubs/pinkbook/pink-appendx.htm#appd. Accessed July 2, 2009; Centers for Disease Control and Prevention (CDC). (2008). Needle length and injection site of intramuscular injections. Available at www.cdc.gov/vaccines/ed/encounter08/Downloads.Table%207.pdf. Accessed June 20, 2009; Centers for Disease Control and Prevention (CDC). (2007). National immunization program. Vaccine administration. (Slide presentation). Available at www.cdc.gov/vaccines/ed/vpd2007/download/slides/admin-images.ppt. Accessed June 23, 2009; and Nicoll, L., & Hesby, A. (2002). Intramuscular injection: An integrative research review and guideline for evidence-based practice. *Applied Nursing Research*, 16(2), 149–162.)

TABLE · 8-2   INTRAMUSCULAR SITE SELECTION

	Recommended Site
Age of Patient	
Infants	Vastus lateralis
Toddlers and children	Vastus lateralis or deltoid
Adults	Ventrogluteal or deltoid
Medication Type	
Biologicals (infants and young children)	Vastus lateralis
Biologicals (older children and adults)	Deltoid
Hepatitis B/Rabies	Deltoid
Medications that are known to be irritating, viscous, or oily solutions	Ventrogluteal

(Adapted from Centers for Disease Control and Prevention (CDC). (2009). *The pink book*: Appendices. Epidemiology and prevention of vaccine preventable diseases. (11th ed.). Appendix D. Vaccine administration. Vaccine administration guidelines. Available www.cdc.gov/vaccines/pubs/pinkbook/pink-appendx.htm#appd. Accessed July 2, 2009; Centers for Disease Control and Prevention (CDC). (2008). Needle length and injection site of intramuscular injections. Available at www.cdc.gov/vaccines/ed/encounter08/Downloads.Table%207.pdf. Accessed June 20, 2009; Centers for Disease Control and Prevention (CDC). (2007). National immunization program. Vaccine administration. (Slide presentation). Available at www.cdc.gov/vaccines/ed/vpd2007/download/slides/admin-images.ppt. Accessed June 23, 2009; and Nicoll, L., & Hesby, A. (2002). Intramuscular injection: An integrative research review and guideline for evidence-based practice. *Applied Nursing Research*, 16(2), 149–162.)

TABLE • 8-3 PATIENT POSITIONING	
Injection Site	**Patient Position**
Deltoid	Patient may sit or stand. A child may be held in an adult's lap.
Ventrogluteal	Patient may stand, sit, lie laterally, and lay supine.
Vastus lateralis	Patient may sit or lay supine. Infants and young children may lay supine or be held in an adult's lap.

(Centers for Disease Control and Prevention (CDC). (2009). The pink book: Appendices. *Epidemiology and prevention of vaccine preventable diseases*. (11th ed.). Appendix D. Vaccine administration. Vaccine administration guidelines. Available www.cedc.gov/vaccines/pubs/pinkbook/pink-appendx.htm#appd. Accessed July 2, 2009.)

ensures it is given using an angle of injection between 72 and 90 degrees (Nicoll & Hesby, 2002). Figure 5-1 in the chapter opener shows the angles of insertion for intramuscular injections.

The volume of medication that can be administered intramuscularly varies based on the intended site. Generally, 1 to 4 mL is the accepted volume range, with no more than 1 to 2 mL given at the deltoid site. The less-developed muscles of children and elderly people limit the intramuscular injection to 1 to 2 mL.

A previously included practice associated with intramuscular injections is the inclusion of aspiration; the process of pulling back on the plunger of the syringe before injection to ensure the medication is not injected into a blood vessel. According to the CDC (2009), aspiration is not required.

EQUIPMENT
- Disposable gloves
- Additional PPE, as indicated
- Medication
- Sterile syringe and needle of appropriate size and gauge
- Antimicrobial swab
- Small gauze square
- Computer-generated Medication Administration Record (CMAR) or Medication Administration Record (MAR)

ASSESSMENT
Assess the patient for any allergies. Check the expiration date before administering medication. Assess the appropriateness of the drug for the patient. Verify patient name, dose, route, and time of administration. Review assessment and laboratory data that may influence drug administration. Assess the site on the patient where the injection is to be given. Avoid any site that is bruised, tender, hard, swollen, inflamed, or scarred.

Assess the patient's knowledge of the medication. If the patient has deficient knowledge about the medication, this may be the appropriate time to begin education about it. If the medication may affect the patient's vital signs, assess them before administration. If the medication is intended for pain relief, assess the patient's pain before and after administration.

NURSING DIAGNOSIS
Determine related factors for the nursing diagnoses based on the patient's current status. Appropriate diagnoses may include:
- Deficient Knowledge
- Risk for Allergy Response
- Risk for Injury
- Acute Pain
- Anxiety

OUTCOME IDENTIFICATION AND PLANNING
The expected outcome to achieve when administering an intramuscular injection is that the patient receives the medication via the intramuscular route. Other outcomes that may be appropriate include the following: the patient's anxiety is decreased; the patient does not experience adverse effects; and the patient understands and complies with the medication regimen.

(continued)

Skill · 8   Administering an Intramuscular Injection   *continued*

IMPLEMENTATION

ACTION	RATIONALE
1. Gather equipment. Check each medication order against the original order in the medical record according to facility policy. Clarify any inconsistencies. Check the patient's chart for allergies.	This comparison helps to identify errors that may have occurred when orders were transcribed. The primary care provider's order is the legal record of medication orders for each facility.
2. Know the actions, special nursing considerations, safe dose ranges, purpose of administration, and adverse effects of the medications to be administered. Consider the appropriateness of the medication for this patient.	This knowledge aids the nurse in evaluating the therapeutic effect of the medication in relation to the patient's disorder and can also be used to educate the patient about the medication.
3. Perform hand hygiene.	Hand hygiene prevents the spread of microorganisms.
4. Move the medication cart to the outside of the patient's room or prepare for administration in the medication area.	Organization facilitates error-free administration and saves time.
5. Unlock the medication cart or drawer. Enter pass code and scan employee identification, if required.	Locking the cart or drawer safeguards each patient's medication supply. Hospital accrediting organizations require medication carts to be locked when not in use. Entering pass code and scanning ID allows only authorized users into the system and identifies user for documentation by the computer.
6. **Prepare medications for one patient at a time.**	This prevents errors in medication administration.
7. Read the CMAR/MAR and select the proper medication from the patient's medication drawer or unit stock.	This is the *first* check of the label.
8. Compare the label with the CMAR/MAR. Check expiration dates and perform calculations, if necessary. Scan the bar code on the package, if required.	This is the *second* check of the label. Verify calculations with another nurse to ensure safety, if necessary.
9. If necessary, withdraw medication from an ampule or vial as described in Skills 5-3 and 5-4.	
10. **When all medications for one patient have been prepared, recheck the label with the MAR before taking the medications to the patient.**	This is a *third* check to ensure accuracy and to prevent errors. Some facilities require the third check to occur at the bedside, after identifying the patient and before administration.
11. Lock the medication cart before leaving it.	Locking the cart or drawer safeguards the patient's medication supply. Hospital accrediting organizations require medication carts to be locked when not in use.
12. Transport medications to the patient's bedside carefully, and keep the medications in sight at all times.	Careful handling and close observation prevent accidental or deliberate disarrangement of medications.
13. **Ensure that the patient receives the medications at the correct time.**	Check agency policy, which may allow for administration within a period of 30 minutes before or 30 minutes after designated time.
14. Perform hand hygiene and put on PPE, if indicated.	Hand hygiene and PPE prevent the spread of microorganisms. PPE is required based on transmission precautions.
15. Identify the patient. Usually, the patient should be identified using two methods. Compare information with the CMAR/MAR.	Identifying the patient ensures the right patient receives the medications and helps prevent errors.
a. Check the name and identification number on the patient's identification band.	This is the most reliable method. Replace the identification band if it is missing or inaccurate in any way.
b. Ask the patient to state his or her name and birth date, based on facility policy.	This requires a response from the patient, but illness and strange surroundings often cause patients to be confused.

ACTION	RATIONALE
c. If the patient cannot identify him- or herself, verify the patient's identification with a staff member who knows the patient for the second source.	This is another way to double-check identity. Do not use the name on the door or over the bed, because these signs may be inaccurate.
16. Close the door to the room or pull the bedside curtain.	This provides patient privacy.
17. Complete necessary assessments before administering medications. Check the patient's allergy bracelet or ask the patient about allergies. Explain the purpose and action of the medication to the patient.	Assessment is a prerequisite to administration of medications. Explanation provides rationale, increases knowledge, and reduces anxiety.
18. Scan the patient's bar code on the identification band, if required.	Provides an additional check to ensure that the medication is given to the right patient.
19. Put on clean gloves.	Gloves help prevent exposure to contaminants.
20. Select an appropriate administration site.	Selecting the appropriate site prevents injury.
21. Assist the patient to the appropriate position for the site chosen. See Table 5-3. Drape, as needed, to expose only the area of site being used.	Appropriate positioning for the site chosen prevents injury. Draping helps maintain the patient's privacy.
22. Identify the appropriate landmarks for the site chosen.	Good visualization is necessary to establish the correct location of the site and to avoid damage to tissues.
23. Cleanse the area around the injection site with an antimicrobial swab. Use a firm, circular motion while moving outward from the injection site. Allow area to dry.	Pathogens on the skin can be forced into the tissues by the needle. Moving from the center outward prevents contamination of the site. Allowing skin to dry prevents introducing alcohol into the tissue, which can be irritating and uncomfortable.
24. Remove the needle cap by pulling it straight off. Hold the syringe in your dominant hand between the thumb and forefinger.	This technique lessens the risk of an accidental needlestick and also prevents inadvertently unscrewing the needle from the barrel of the syringe.
25. Displace the skin in a Z-track manner by pulling the skin down or to one side about 1 inch (2.5 cm) with your nondominant hand and hold the skin and tissue in this position (Figure 2). (See the accompanying Skill Variation for information on administering an intramuscular injection without using the Z-track technique.)	This ensures medication does not leak back along the needle track and into the subcutaneous tissue.

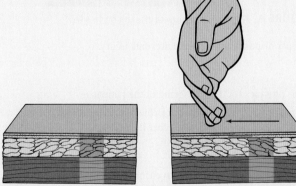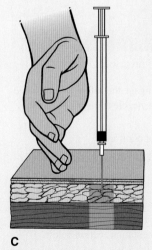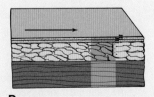

A   B   C   D

FIGURE 2. The Z-track or zigzag technique is recommended for intramuscular injections. (**A**) Normal skin and tissues. (**B**) Moving the skin to one side. (**C**) Needle is inserted at a 90-degree angle, and the nurse aspirates for blood. (**D**) Once the needle is withdrawn, displaced tissue is allowed to return to its normal position, preventing the solution from escaping from the muscle tissue.

(continued)

Skill · 8 **Administering an Intramuscular Injection** *continued*

ACTION

RATIONALE

26. Quickly dart the needle into the tissue so that the needle is perpendicular to the patient's body (Figure 3). This should ensure that it is given using an angle of injection between 72 and 90 degrees.

A quick injection is less painful. Inserting the needle at a 72- to 90-degree angle facilitates entry into muscle tissue.

27. As soon as the needle is in place, use the thumb and forefinger of your nondominant hand to hold the lower end of the syringe. Slide your dominant hand to the end of the plunger. Inject the solution slowly (10 sec/mL of medication).

Moving the syringe could cause damage to the tissues and inadvertent administration into incorrect area. Rapid injection of the solution creates pressure in the tissues, resulting in discomfort. An outdated practice is the inclusion of aspiration (process of pulling back on the plunger of the syringe before injection to ensure the medication is not injected into a blood vessel) has been part of this procedure in the past. According to the CDC (2009), this procedure is not required.

28. Once the medication has been instilled, wait 10 seconds before withdrawing the needle.

Allows medication to begin to diffuse into the surrounding muscle tissue (Nicoll & Hesby, 2002).

29. Withdraw the needle smoothly and steadily at the same angle at which it was inserted, supporting tissue around the injection site with your nondominant hand.

Slow withdrawal of the needle pulls the tissues and causes discomfort. Applying counter traction around the injection site helps to prevent pulling on the tissue as the needle is withdrawn. Removing the needle at the same angle at which it was inserted minimizes tissue damage and discomfort for the patient.

30. **Apply gentle pressure at the site with a dry gauze (Figure 4).** Do not massage the site.

Light pressure causes less trauma and irritation to the tissues. Massaging can force medication into subcutaneous tissues.

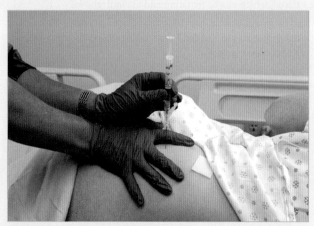

FIGURE 3. Darting the needle into the tissue.

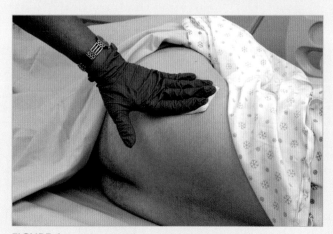

FIGURE 4. Applying pressure at the injection site.

31. Do not recap the used needle. Engage the safety shield or needle guard, if present. Discard the needle and syringe in the appropriate receptacle.

Proper disposal of the needle prevents injury.

32. Assist the patient to a position of comfort.

This provides for the well-being of the patient.

 33. Remove gloves and additional PPE, if used. Perform hand hygiene.

Removing PPE properly reduces the risk for infection transmission and contamination of other items. Hand hygiene prevents the spread of microorganisms.

34. Document the administration of the medication immediately after administration. See Documentation section below.

Timely documentation helps to ensure patient safety.

35. Evaluate the patient's response to medication within an appropriate time frame. Assess site, if possible, within 2 to 4 hours after administration.

The patient needs to be evaluated for therapeutic and adverse effects from the medication. Visualization of the site allows for assessment of any untoward effects.

EVALUATION

The expected outcomes are met when the patient receives the medication via the intramuscular route; the patient's anxiety is decreased; the patient does not experience adverse effects or injury; and the patient understands and complies with the medication regimen.

DOCUMENTATION
Guidelines

Record each medication given on the CMAR/MAR or record using the required format, including date, time, and the site of administration, immediately after administration. If using a bar-code system, medication administration is automatically recorded when the bar code is scanned. PRN medications require documentation of the reason for administration. Prompt recording avoids the possibility of accidentally repeating the administration of the drug. If the drug was refused or omitted, record this in the appropriate area on the medication record and notify the primary care provider. This verifies the reason medication was omitted and ensures that the primary care provider is aware of the patient's condition.

UNEXPECTED SITUATIONS AND ASSOCIATED INTERVENTIONS

- *You stick yourself with needle before injection:* Discard needle and syringe appropriately. Follow agency policy regarding needlestick injury. Prepare new syringe with medication and administer to patient. Complete appropriate paperwork and follow facility's policy regarding accidental needlesticks.
- *You stick yourself with needle after injection:* Discard needle and syringe appropriately. Follow agency policy regarding needlestick injury. Complete appropriate paperwork and follow facility's policy regarding accidental needlesticks.
- *During injection, patient pulls away from needle before medication is delivered fully:* Remove and appropriately discard needle. Attach a new needle to syringe and administer remaining medication at a different site. Document events and interventions, according to facility policy.
- *While injecting needle into patient, you hit patient's bone:* Withdraw and discard the needle. Apply new needle to syringe and administer in alternate site. Document incident in patient's medical record. Notify primary care provider. Complete appropriate paperwork related to special events according to facility policy.

SPECIAL CONSIDERATIONS
General Considerations

- Ongoing assessment is an important part of nursing care for both evaluation of patient response to administered medications and early detection of adverse effects. If an adverse effect is suspected, withhold further medication doses and notify the patient's primary healthcare provider. Additional intervention is based on the type of reaction and patient assessment.

Infant and Child Considerations

- The vastus lateralis is the preferred site for infants.

Older Adult Considerations

- Muscle mass atrophies as a person ages. Take care to evaluate the patient's muscle mass and body composition. Use appropriate needle length and gauge for patient's body composition. Choose appropriate site based on the patient's body composition.

Home Care Considerations

- Encourage patients to consult the policies of their local government regarding contaminated and sharps waste disposal. Explain that needles and syringes should be disposed of in a hard, plastic container. Liquid detergent or liquid fabric softener containers are good choices. Glass containers should not be used.

(continued)

Skill · 8   Administering an Intramuscular Injection   *continued*

Skill Variation   Administering an Intramuscular Injection Without Using the Z-Track Technique

If the Z-Track technique is not used, stretch the skin flat between two fingers and hold it taut for needle insertion. To administer the injection:

1. Perform hand hygiene and put on PPE, as indicated.

2. Identify the patient.

3. Explain procedure to patient.

4. Select an appropriate administration site.

5. Assist the patient to the appropriate position for the site chosen. Drape, as needed, to expose only area of site to be used.

6. Put on gloves.

7. Identify the appropriate landmarks for the site chosen with your nondominant hand.

8. Clean the area around the injection site with an antimicrobial swab. Use a firm, circular motion while moving outward from the injection site. Allow area to dry.

9. Remove the needle cap by pulling it straight off. Hold the syringe in your dominant hand between the thumb and forefinger.

10. Stretch the skin flat between two fingers and hold taut for needle insertion.

11. Quickly dart the needle into the tissue so that the needle is perpendicular to the patient's body. This should ensure that it is given using an angle of injection between 72 and 90 degrees.

12. As soon as the needle is in place, use your thumb and forefinger of your nondominant hand to hold the lower end of the syringe. Slide your dominant hand to the end of the plunger.

13. Inject the solution slowly (10 sec/mL of medication).

14. Withdraw the needle smoothly and steadily at the same angle at which it was inserted, supporting tissue around the injection site with your nondominant hand.

15. Apply gentle pressure at the site with a dry gauze.

16. Do not recap the used needle. Engage the safety shield or needle guard. Discard the needle and syringe in the appropriate receptacle.

17. Assist the patient to a position of comfort.

18. Remove gloves and additional PPE, if used. Perform hand hygiene.

19. Document administration of the medication on the CMAR/MAR immediately after performing the procedure.

20. Evaluate the patient's response to medication within an appropriate time frame. Assess site, if possible, within 2 to 4 hours after administration.

Skill · 9   Administering Continuous Subcutaneous Infusion: Applying an Insulin Pump

Some medications, such as insulin and morphine, may be administered continuously via the subcutaneous route. Continuous subcutaneous insulin infusion (CSII or insulin pump) allows for multiple preset rates of insulin delivery. This system uses a small, computerized reservoir that delivers insulin via tubing through a needle inserted into the subcutaneous tissue. The pump is programmed to deliver multiple preset rates of insulin delivery. The settings can be adjusted for exercise and illness, and bolus dose delivery can be timed in relation to meals. Change sites every 2 to 3 days to prevent tissue damage or absorption problems (Olohan & Zappitelli, 2003). Advantages of continuous subcutaneous medication infusion include the longer rate of absorption via the subcutaneous route and convenience for the patient.

EQUIPMENT	• Insulin pump • Pump syringe and vial of insulin or prefilled cartridge, as ordered • Sterile infusion set • Insertion (triggering) device • Needle (24 or 22 gauge, or blunt-ended needle) • Antimicrobial swabs • Sterile nonocclusive dressing • Computer-generated Medication Administration Record (CMAR) or Medication Administration Record (MAR) • Clean gloves • Additional PPE, as indicated

---

ASSESSMENT

Assess the patient for any allergies. Check the expiration date before administering medication. Assess the appropriateness of the drug for the patient. Review assessment and laboratory data that may influence drug administration. Verify patient name, dose, route, and time of administration. Assess the infusion site. Typical infusion sites include those areas used for subcutaneous insulin injection. Assess the area where the pump is to be applied. Do not place the pump on skin that is irritated or broken down.

Assess the patient's knowledge of the medication. If the patient has a knowledge deficit about the medication, this may be the appropriate time to begin education about it. Assess the patient's blood glucose level as appropriate or as ordered.

NURSING DIAGNOSIS

Determine related factors for the nursing diagnoses based on the patient's current status. Appropriate nursing diagnoses may include:
- Deficient Knowledge
- Risk for Impaired Skin Integrity
- Risk for Infection
- Risk for Allergy Response
- Acute Pain

OUTCOME IDENTIFICATION AND PLANNING

The expected outcome is that the device is applied successfully and medication is administered. Other outcomes that may be appropriate include the following: patient understands the rationale for the pump use and mechanism of action; patient experiences no allergy response; patient's skin remains intact; pump is applied using aseptic technique; and patient does not experience adverse effect.

IMPLEMENTATION

ACTION	**RATIONALE**
1. Gather equipment. Check each medication order against the original order in the medical record, according to facility policy. Clarify any inconsistencies. Check the patient's chart for allergies.	This comparison helps to identify errors that may have occurred when orders were transcribed. The primary care provider's order is the legal record of medication orders for each facility.
2. Know the actions, special nursing considerations, safe dose ranges, purpose of administration, and adverse effects of the medications to be administered. Consider the appropriateness of the medication for this patient.	This knowledge aids the nurse in evaluating the therapeutic effect of the medication in relation to the patient's disorder and can also be used to educate the patient about the medication.
3. Perform hand hygiene.	Hand hygiene prevents the spread of microorganisms.
4. Move the medication cart to the outside of the patient's room or prepare for administration in the medication area.	Organization facilitates error-free administration and saves time.
5. Unlock the medication cart or drawer. Enter pass code and scan employee identification, if required.	Locking the cart or drawer safeguards each patient's medication supply. Hospital accrediting organizations require medication carts to be locked when not in use. Entering pass code and scanning ID allows only authorized users into the system and identifies user for documentation by the computer.

(continued)

Skill · 9   Administering Continuous Subcutaneous Infusion: Applying an Insulin Pump *continued*

ACTION	RATIONALE
6. **Prepare medications for one patient at a time.**	This prevents errors in medication administration.
7. Read the CMAR/MAR and select the proper medication from the patient's medication drawer or unit stock.	This is the *first* check of the label.
8. Compare the label with the CMAR/MAR. Check expiration dates and perform calculations, if necessary. Scan the bar code on the package, if required.	This is the *second* check of the label. Verify calculations with another nurse to ensure safety, if necessary.
9. Attach a blunt-ended needle or a small-gauge needle to a syringe. Follow Skill 5-4 to remove insulin from vial, if necessary. Remove enough insulin to last patient 2 to 3 days, plus 30 units for priming tubing. If using prepackaged insulin syringe or cartridge, remove from packaging.	Patient will wear pump for up to 3 days without changing syringe or tubing.
10. **When all medications for one patient have been prepared, recheck the label with the MAR before taking them to the patient.**	This is a *third* check to ensure accuracy and to prevent errors. Some facilities require the third check to occur at the bedside, after identifying the patient and before administration.
11. Lock the medication cart before leaving it.	Locking the cart or drawer safeguards the patient's medication supply. Hospital accrediting organizations require medication carts to be locked when not in use.
12. Transport medications to the patient's bedside carefully, and keep the medications in sight at all times.	Careful handling and close observation prevent accidental or deliberate disarrangement of medications.
13. **Ensure that the patient receives the medications at the correct time.**	Check agency policy, which may allow for administration within a period of 30 minutes before or 30 minutes after designated time.
14. Perform hand hygiene and put on PPE, if indicated.	Hand hygiene and PPE prevent the spread of microorganisms. PPE is required based on transmission precautions.
15. Identify the patient. Usually, the patient should be identified using two methods. Compare information with the CMAR/MAR.	Identifying the patient ensures the right patient receives the medications and helps prevent errors.
a. Check the name and identification number on the patient's identification band.	This is the most reliable method. Replace the identification band if it is missing or inaccurate in any way.
b. Ask the patient to state his or her name and birth date, based on facility policy.	This requires a response from the patient, but illness and strange surroundings often cause patients to be confused.
c. If the patient cannot identify him- or herself, verify the patient's identification with a staff member who knows the patient.	This is another way to double-check identity. Do not use the name on the door or over the bed, because these signs may be inaccurate.
16. Close the door to the room or pull the bedside curtain.	This provides patient privacy.
17. Complete necessary assessments before administering medications. Check the patient's allergy bracelet or ask the patient about allergies. Explain the purpose and action of the medication to the patient.	Assessment is a prerequisite to administration of medications. Explanation provides rationale, increases knowledge, and reduces anxiety.
18. Scan the patient's bar code on the identification band, if required.	Provides an additional check to ensure that the medication is given to the right patient.
19. Perform hand hygiene. Put on gloves.	Hand hygiene prevents the spread of microorganisms. Gloves prevent contact with blood and body fluids.
20. Remove the cap from the syringe or insulin cartridge (Figure 1). Attach sterile tubing to syringe or insulin cartridge. Open the pump and place the syringe or cartridge in compartment according to manufacturer's directions (Figure 2). Close the pump.	Removing all air from the tubing ensures that the patient receives the correct dose of insulin.

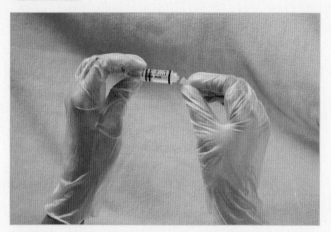

FIGURE 1. Removing the cap from the syringe or insulin cartridge.

21. Initiate priming of the tubing, according to manufacturer's directions. Program the pump according to manufacturer's recommendations following primary care provider's orders (Figure 3). **Check for any bubbles in the tubing.**

22. Activate the delivery device. Place the needle between prongs of the insertion device with the sharp edge facing out. Push insertion set down until a click is heard.

23. Select an appropriate administration site.

24. Assist the patient to the appropriate position for the site chosen. Drape, as needed, to expose only area of site to be used.

25. Identify the appropriate landmarks for the site chosen.

26. Cleanse area around injection site with antimicrobial swab (Figure 4). Use a firm, circular motion while moving outward from insertion site. Allow antiseptic to dry.

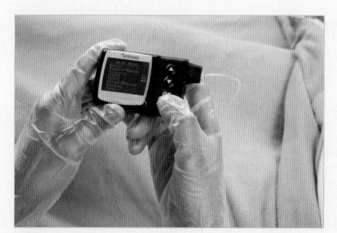

FIGURE 3. Programming the pump according to manufacturer's recommendations following primary care provider's orders.

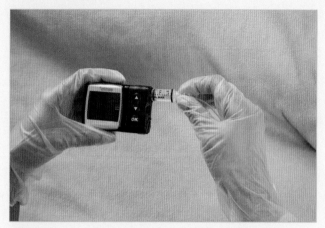

FIGURE 2. Placing the syringe or cartridge in compartment according to manufacturer's directions.

Syringe must be placed in pump correctly for delivery of insulin.

To ensure correct placement of insulin pump needle, an insertion device must be used.

Appropriate site prevents injury.

Appropriate site prevents injury. Draping maintains privacy and warmth.

Good visualization is necessary to establish the correct location of the site and avoid damage to tissues.

Pathogens on the skin can be forced into the tissues by the needle. Moving from the center outward prevents contamination of the site. Allowing skin to dry prevents introducing alcohol into the tissue, which can be irritating and uncomfortable.

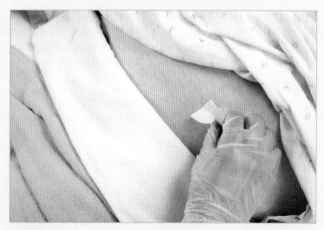

FIGURE 4. Cleansing area around injection site with antimicrobial swab.

(continued)

Skill · 9 — Administering Continuous Subcutaneous Infusion: Applying an Insulin Pump *continued*

ACTION

RATIONALE

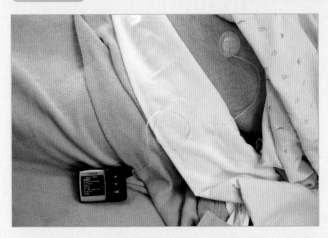

FIGURE 5. Insulin pump in place.

27. Remove paper from adhesive backing. Remove the needle guard. Pinch skin at insertion site, press insertion device on site, and press release button to insert needle. Remove triggering device.

To ensure delivery of insulin into subcutaneous tissue, a skin fold is made with a pinch *before* insertion of the medication.

28. Apply sterile occlusive dressing over insertion site, if not part of insertion device. Attach the pump to patient's clothing, as desired (Figure 5).

Dressing prevents contamination of site. Pump can be dislodged easily if not attached securely to patient.

29. Assist the patient to a position of comfort.

This provides for the well-being of the patient.

30. Discard the needle and syringe in the appropriate receptacle.

Proper disposal of the needle prevents injury.

31. Remove gloves and additional PPE, if used. Perform hand hygiene.

Removing PPE properly reduces the risk for infection transmission and contamination of other items. Hand hygiene prevents the spread of microorganisms.

32. Document the administration of the medication immediately after administration. See Documentation section below.

Timely documentation helps to ensure patient safety.

33. Evaluate the patient's response to medication within appropriate time frame. Monitor the patient's blood glucose levels, as appropriate, or as ordered.

Patient needs to be evaluated to ensure that pump is delivering drug appropriately. The patient needs to be evaluated for therapeutic and adverse effects from the medication.

EVALUATION

The expected outcomes are met when the patient receives insulin from the attached pump successfully without hypo- or hyperglycemic effects noted; patient understands the rationale for the pump attachment; patient experiences no allergy response; patient's skin remains intact; patient remains infection free; and patient experiences no or minimal pain.

DOCUMENTATION

Guidelines

Document the application of the pump, the type of insulin used, pump settings, insertion site, and any teaching done with patient on the CMAR/MAR or record using the required format, including date, time, and the site of administration, immediately after administration. If using a bar-code system, medication administration is automatically recorded when the bar code is scanned. PRN medications require documentation of the reason for administration. Prompt recording avoids the possibility of accidentally repeating the administration of the drug. If the drug was refused or omitted, record this in the appropriate area on the medication record and notify the primary care provider. This verifies the reason medication was omitted and ensures that the primary care provider is aware of the patient's condition.

Sample Documentation

> 9/22/12 1000 Insulin pump inserted by patient on left upper quadrant of abdomen with minimal assistance. Pump filled with 300 units (3 mL) of lispro insulin. Rate set at 1 unit per hour. Patient verbalizes desire to apply pump without assistance when site next changed.
>
> —B. Clapp, RN

UNEXPECTED SITUATIONS AND ASSOCIATED INTERVENTIONS

- *After the pump is attached to patient, a large amount of air is noted in tubing:* Remove the pump from patient. Obtain new sterile tubing with insertion needle. Prime the tubing and reinsert.
- *Patient must rotate site more frequently than every 2 to 3 days due to insulin usage:* Check manufacturer's recommendations. Most pumps are initially set in a smaller mode but can be changed for a large amount of insulin delivery.
- *Patient is refusing to rotate site at least every 3 days:* Inform the patient that absorption of medication decreases after 3 days, which may increase his or her need for insulin. Rotating sites prevents this decrease in absorption from developing. In addition, rotation of sites reduces risk of infection at site.
- *You note that insertion site is now erythematous:* Remove the stylet, obtain a new pump setup, and insert at a different site at least 1 inch from old site.
- *Occlusive dressing will not stick due to perspiration:* Apply deodorant around insertion site but not over insertion site. Alternately, apply skin barrier around insertion site but not over insertion site.

SPECIAL CONSIDERATIONS
General Considerations

- Assess infusion site areas routinely for inflammation, allergic reactions, infection, and lipodystrophy.
- Good hygiene and frequent catheter site changes reduce risk of site complications. Change catheter site every 2 to 3 days.
- Contact dermatitis is sometimes a problem at the catheter site area. The primary care provider may order topical antibiotics, aloe, vitamin E, or corticosteroids to treat a contact dermatitis.
- Insulin self-administered by the patient through the insulin pump should be communicated to the nurse at the time of administration. This allows for accurate documentation of insulin requirements.
- Ongoing assessment is an important part of nursing care for both evaluation of patient response to administered medications and early detection of adverse effects. If an adverse effect is suspected, withhold further medication doses and notify the patient's primary healthcare provider. Additional intervention is based on type of reaction and patient assessment.

Home Care Considerations

- Encourage patients to consult the policies of their local government regarding contaminated and sharps waste disposal. Explain that needles and other sharps should be disposed of in a hard, plastic container. Liquid detergent or liquid fabric softener containers are good choices. Glass containers should not be used.

Skill · 10 Administering Medications by Intravenous Bolus or Push Through an Intravenous Infusion

A medication can be administered as an IV bolus or push. This involves a single injection of a concentrated solution directly into an IV line. Drugs given by IV push are used for intermittent dosing or to treat emergencies. The drug is administered very slowly over at least 1 minute. This can be done manually or a syringe pump may be used. Confirm exact administration times by consulting a pharmacist or drug reference.

(continued)

Skill · 10 **Administering Medications by Intravenous Bolus or Push Through an Intravenous Infusion** *continued*

EQUIPMENT	
	• Antimicrobial swab
• Watch with second hand, or stopwatch
• Clean gloves
• Additional PPE, as indicated
• Prescribed medication
• Syringe with a needleless device or 23- to 25-gauge, 1-inch needle (follow facility policy)
• Syringe pump, if necessary
• Computer-generated Medication Administration Record (CMAR) or Medication Administration Record (MAR)

ASSESSMENT

Assess the patient for any allergies. Check the expiration date before administering medication. Assess the appropriateness of the drug for the patient. Assess the compatibility of the ordered medication and the IV fluid. Review assessment and laboratory data that may influence drug administration. Verify the patient's name, dose, route, and time of administration. Assess patient's IV site, noting any swelling, coolness, leakage of fluid from the IV site, or pain. Assess the patient's knowledge of the medication.

If the patient has a knowledge deficit about the medication, this may be the appropriate time to begin education about the medication. If the medication may affect the patient's vital signs, assess them before administration. If the medication is for pain relief, assess the patient's pain before and after administration.

NURSING DIAGNOSIS

Determine related factors for the nursing diagnoses based on the patient's current status. Appropriate nursing diagnoses may include:

- Acute Pain
- Deficient Knowledge
- Risk for Injury
- Risk for Allergy Response
- Risk for Infection
- Anxiety

OUTCOME IDENTIFICATION AND PLANNING

The expected outcome to achieve is that the medication is given safely via the **intravenous route**. Other outcomes that may be appropriate include the following: patient experiences no adverse effect; patient experiences no allergy response; patient is knowledgeable about medication being added by bolus IV; patient remains infection free; and patient has no, or decreased, anxiety.

IMPLEMENTATION

ACTION

RATIONALE

1. Gather equipment. Check medication order against the original order in the medical record, according to facility policy. Clarify any inconsistencies. Check the patient's chart for allergies. Verify the compatibility of the medication and IV fluid. Check a drug resource to clarify whether the medication needs to be diluted before administration. Check the infusion rate.

This comparison helps to identify errors that may have occurred when orders were transcribed. The primary care provider's order is the legal record of medication orders for each facility. Compatibility of medication and solution prevents complications. Delivers the correct dose of medication as prescribed.

2. Know the actions, special nursing considerations, safe dose ranges, purpose of administration, and adverse effects of the medications to be administered. Consider the appropriateness of the medication for this patient.

This knowledge aids the nurse in evaluating the therapeutic effect of the medication in relation to the patient's disorder and can also be used to educate the patient about the medication.

3. Perform hand hygiene.

Hand hygiene prevents the spread of microorganisms.

4. Move the medication cart to the outside of the patient's room or prepare for administration in the medication area.

Organization facilitates error-free administration and saves time.

5. Unlock the medication cart or drawer. Enter pass code and scan employee identification, if required.

Locking the cart or drawer safeguards each patient's medication supply. Hospital accrediting organizations require medication carts to be locked when not in use. Entering pass code and scanning ID allows only authorized users into the system and identifies user for documentation by the computer.

ACTION	RATIONALE
6. **Prepare medication for one patient at a time.**	This prevents errors in medication administration.
7. Read the CMAR/MAR and select the proper medication from the patient's medication drawer or unit stock.	This is the *first* check of the label.
8. Compare the label with the CMAR/MAR. Check expiration dates and perform calculations, if necessary. Scan the bar code on the package, if required.	This is the *second* check of the label. Verify calculations with another nurse to ensure safety, if necessary.
9. If necessary, withdraw medication from an ampule or vial as described in Skills 5-3 and 5-4.	
10. **Recheck the label with the MAR before taking it to the patient.**	This is a *third* check to ensure accuracy and to prevent errors. Some facilities require the third check to occur at the bedside, after identifying the patient and before administration.
11. Lock the medication cart before leaving it.	Locking the cart or drawer safeguards the patient's medication supply. Hospital accrediting organizations require medication carts to be locked when not in use.
12. Transport medications and equipment to the patient's bedside carefully, and keep the medications in sight at all times.	Careful handling and close observation prevent accidental or deliberate disarrangement of medications. Having equipment available saves time and facilitates performance of the task.
13. **Ensure that the patient receives the medications at the correct time.**	Check agency policy, which may allow for administration within a period of 30 minutes before or 30 minutes after designated time.
14. Perform hand hygiene and put on PPE, if indicated.	Hand hygiene and PPE prevent the spread of microorganisms. PPE is required based on transmission precautions.
15. Identify the patient. Usually, the patient should be identified using two methods. Compare information with the CMAR/MAR.	Identifying the patient ensures the right patient receives the medications and helps prevent errors.
a. Check the name and identification number on the patient's identification band.	This is the most reliable method. Replace the identification band if it is missing or inaccurate in any way.
b. Ask the patient to state his or her name and birth date, based on facility policy.	This requires a response from the patient, but illness and strange surroundings often cause patients to be confused.
c. If the patient cannot identify him- or herself, verify the patient's identification with a staff member who knows the patient for the second source.	This is another way to double-check identity. Do not use the name on the door or over the bed, because these signs may be inaccurate.
16. Close the door to the room or pull the bedside curtain.	This provides patient privacy.
17. Complete necessary assessments before administering medications. Check the patient's allergy bracelet or ask the patient about allergies. Explain the purpose and action of the medication to the patient.	Assessment is a prerequisite to administration of medications. Explanation provides rationale, increases knowledge, and reduces anxiety.
18. Scan the patient's bar code on the identification band, if required.	Provides an additional check to ensure that the medication is given to the right patient.
19. **Assess IV site for presence of inflammation or infiltration.**	IV medication must be given directly into a vein for safe administration.
20. If IV infusion is being administered via an infusion pump, pause the pump.	Pausing prevents infusion of fluid during bolus administration and activation of pump occlusion alarms.
21. Put on clean gloves.	Gloves prevent contact with blood and body fluids.
22. Select injection port on tubing that is closest to venipuncture site. Clean port with antimicrobial swab.	Using port closest to needle insertion site minimizes dilution of medication. Cleaning deters entry of microorganisms when port is punctured.

(continued)

Skill · 10 **Administering Medications by Intravenous Bolus or Push Through an Intravenous Infusion** *continued*

ACTION

23. Uncap syringe. Steady port with your nondominant hand while inserting syringe into center of port.

24. Move your nondominant hand to the section of IV tubing just above the injection port. Fold the tubing between your fingers.

25. Pull back slightly on plunger just until blood appears in tubing.

26. **Inject the medication at the recommended rate** (see Special Considerations below) (Figure 1).

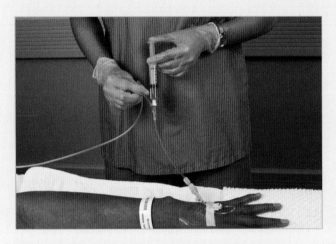

RATIONALE

This supports the injection port and lessens the risk for accidentally dislodging the IV or entering the port incorrectly.

This temporarily stops flow of gravity IV infusion and prevents medication from backing up tubing.

This ensures injection of medication into the bloodstream.

This delivers correct amount of medication at proper interval according to manufacturer's directions.

FIGURE 1. Injecting medication while interrupting IV flow. *(Photo by B. Proud.)*

27. Release the tubing. Remove the syringe. Do not recap the used needle, if used. Engage the safety shield or needle guard, if present. Release the tubing and allow the IV fluid to flow. Discard the needle and syringe in the appropriate receptacle.

28. Check IV fluid infusion rate. Restart infusion pump, if appropriate.

 29. Remove gloves and additional PPE, if used. Perform hand hygiene.

30. Document the administration of the medication immediately after administration. See Documentation section below.

31. Evaluate the patient's response to medication within appropriate time frame.

Proper disposal of the needle prevents injury.

Injection of bolus may alter rate of fluid infusion, if infusing by gravity.

Removing PPE properly reduces the risk for infection transmission and contamination of other items. Hand hygiene prevents the spread of microorganisms.

Timely documentation helps to ensure patient safety.

The patient needs to be evaluated for therapeutic and adverse effects from the medication.

EVALUATION

The expected outcomes are met when the medication is safely administered via IV bolus; the patient's anxiety is decreased; the patient does not experience adverse effects; and the patient understands and complies with the medication regimen.

DOCUMENTATION

Guidelines

Document the administration of the medication immediately after administration, including date, time, dose, route of administration, site of administration, and rate of administration on the CMAR/MAR or record using the required format. If using a bar-code system, medication administration is automatically recorded when the bar code is scanned. PRN medications require documentation of the reason for administration. Prompt recording avoids the possibility of accidentally repeating the administration of the drug. If the drug was refused or omitted, record this in the appropriate area on the medication record and notify the primary care provider. This verifies the reason medication was omitted and ensures that the primary care provider is aware of the patient's condition.

UNEXPECTED SITUATIONS AND ASSOCIATED INTERVENTIONS

- *Upon assessing IV site before administering medication, no blood return is aspirated:* If IV appears patent, without signs of infiltration, and IV fluid infuses without difficulty, proceed with administration. Observe closely for signs and symptoms of infiltration during and after administration.
- *Upon assessing patient's IV site before administering medication, you note that IV has infiltrated:* Stop IV fluid and remove IV from extremity. Restart IV in a different location. Continue to monitor new IV site as medication is administered.
- *While administering medication, you note a cloudy, white substance forming in IV tubing:* Stop IV from flowing and stop administering medication. Clamp IV at site nearest to patient. Change administration tubing and restart infusion. Check literature or consult pharmacist regarding compatibility of medication and IV fluid.
- *While you are administering medication, patient begins to complain of pain at IV site:* Stop medication. Assess IV site for any signs of infiltration or phlebitis. Flush the IV with normal saline to check for patency. If the IV site appears within normal limits, resume medication administration at a slower rate.

SPECIAL CONSIDERATIONS

- Facility policy may recommend the following variations when injecting a bolus IV medication:
  - Release folded tubing after each increment of the drug has been administered at prescribed rate to facilitate delivery of medication.
  - Use a syringe with 1 mL normal saline to flush tubing after an IV bolus is delivered to ensure that residual medication in tubing is not delivered too rapidly.
- Consider how fast IV fluid is flowing to determine whether a flush of normal saline is in order after administering medication. If IV fluid is flowing less than 50 mL per hour, it may take medication up to 30 minutes to reach patient. This depends on what type of tubing is being used in the agency.
- If the IV is a small gauge (22- to 24-gauge) placed in a small vein, a blood return may not occur even if IV is intact. Also, patient may complain of stinging and pain at site while medication is being administered due to irritation of vein. Placing a warm pack over the vein or slowing the rate may relieve discomfort.
- If the medication and IV solution are incompatible, a bolus may be given by flushing the tubing with normal saline before and after the medication bolus. Consult facility policy.
- Ongoing assessment is an important part of nursing care for both evaluation of patient response to administered medications and early detection of adverse effects. If an adverse effect is suspected, withhold further medication doses and notify the patient's primary healthcare provider. Additional intervention is based on type of reaction and patient assessment.

Skill · 11   Administering a Piggyback Intermittent Intravenous Infusion of Medication

With intermittent IV infusion, the drug is mixed with a small amount of the IV solution, such as 50 to 100 mL, and administered over a short period at the prescribed interval (e.g., every 4 hours). The administration is most often performed using an IV infusion pump, which requires the nurse to program the infusion rate into the pump. "Smart (computerized) pumps" are being used by many facilities for IV infusions, including intermittent infusions. Smart pumps also require programming of infusion rates by the nurse, but also are able to identify dosing limits and practice guidelines to aid in safe administration. Administration may be achieved by gravity infusion, which requires the nurse to calculate the infusion rate in drops per minute. The best practice, however, is to use an IV infusion pump.

The IV piggyback delivery system requires the intermittent or additive solution to be placed higher than the primary solution container. An extension hook provided by the manufacturer provides for easy lowering of the main IV container. The port on the primary IV line has a back-check valve that automatically stops the flow of the primary solution, allowing the secondary or piggyback solution to flow when connected. Because manufacturers' designs vary, it is important to check the directions carefully for the systems used in the facility. The nurse is responsible for calculating and regulating the infusion with an infusion pump or manually adjusting the flow rate of the IV intermittent infusion.

(continued)

Skill · 11 Administering a Piggyback Intermittent Intravenous Infusion of Medication *continued*

EQUIPMENT	• Medication prepared in labeled small-volume bag • Short secondary infusion tubing (microdrip or macrodrip) • IV pump • Needleless connector, if required, based on facility system • Antimicrobial swab • Metal or plastic hook • IV pole • Date label for tubing • Computer-generated Medication Administration Record (CMAR) or Medication Administration Record (MAR) • PPE, as indicated
ASSESSMENT	Assess the patient for any allergies. Check the expiration date before administering medication. Assess the appropriateness of the drug for the patient. Assess the compatibility of the ordered medication, diluent, and the infusing IV fluid. Review assessment and laboratory data that may influence drug administration. Verify patient name, dose, route, and time of administration. Assess the patient's knowledge of the medication. If the patient has a knowledge deficit about the medication, this may be the appropriate time to begin education about the medication. If the medication may affect the patient's vital signs, assess them before administration. Assess the IV insertion site, noting any swelling, coolness, leakage of fluid at site, redness, or pain.
NURSING DIAGNOSIS	Determine related factors for the nursing diagnoses based on the patient's current status. Appropriate nursing diagnoses include: • Risk for Allergy Response • Risk for Infection • Deficient Knowledge • Risk for Injury
OUTCOME IDENTIFICATION AND PLANNING	The expected outcome to achieve is that the medication is delivered via the intravenous route using sterile technique. Other outcomes that may be appropriate include the following: medication is delivered to the patient in a safe manner and at the appropriate infusion rate; patient experiences no allergy response; patient remains infection free; and the patient understands and complies with the medication regimen.

IMPLEMENTATION

ACTION	RATIONALE
1. Gather equipment. Check each medication order against the original order in the medical record, according to facility policy. Clarify any inconsistencies. Check the patient's chart for allergies.	This comparison helps to identify errors that may have occurred when orders were transcribed. The primary care provider's order is the legal record of medication orders for each facility.
2. Know the actions, special nursing considerations, safe dose ranges, purpose of administration, and adverse effects of the medications to be administered. Consider the appropriateness of the medication for this patient.	This knowledge aids the nurse in evaluating the therapeutic effect of the medication in relation to the patient's disorder and can also be used to educate the patient about the medication.
3. Perform hand hygiene.	Hand hygiene prevents the spread of microorganisms.
4. Move the medication cart to the outside of the patient's room or prepare for administration in the medication area.	Organization facilitates error-free administration and saves time.
5. Unlock the medication cart or drawer. Enter pass code and scan employee identification, if required.	Locking the cart or drawer safeguards each patient's medication supply. Hospital accrediting organizations require medication carts to be locked when not in use. Entering pass code and scanning ID allows only authorized users into the system and identifies user for documentation by the computer.

ACTION	RATIONALE
6. **Prepare medications for one patient at a time.**	This prevents errors in medication administration.
7. Read the CMAR/MAR and select the proper medication from the patient's medication drawer or unit stock.	This is the *first* check of the label.
8. Compare the label with the CMAR/MAR. Check expiration dates. Confirm the prescribed or appropriate infusion rate. Calculate the drip rate if using gravity system. Scan the bar code on the package, if required.	This is the *second* check of the label. Verify calculations with another nurse to ensure safety, if necessary. Infusing medication at appropriate rate prevents injury.
9. **When all medications for one patient have been prepared, recheck the label with the MAR before taking them to the patient.**	This is a *third* check to ensure accuracy and to prevent errors. Some facilities require the third check to occur at the bedside, after identifying the patient and before administration.
10. Lock the medication cart before leaving it.	Locking the cart or drawer safeguards the patient's medication supply. Hospital accrediting organizations require medication carts to be locked when not in use.
11. Transport medications to the patient's bedside carefully, and keep the medications in sight at all times.	Careful handling and close observation prevent accidental or deliberate disarrangement of medications.
12. **Ensure that the patient receives the medications at the correct time.**	Check agency policy, which may allow for administration within a period of 30 minutes before or 30 minutes after designated time.
13. Perform hand hygiene and put on PPE, if indicated.	Hand hygiene and PPE prevent the spread of microorganisms. PPE is required based on transmission precautions.
14. Identify the patient. Usually, the patient should be identified using two methods. Compare information with the CMAR/MAR.	Identifying the patient ensures the right patient receives the medications and helps prevent errors.
a. Check the name and identification number on the patient's identification band.	This is the most reliable method. Replace the identification band if it is missing or inaccurate in any way.
b. Ask the patient to state his or her name and birth date, based on facility policy.	This requires a response from the patient, but illness and strange surroundings often cause patients to be confused.
c. If the patient cannot identify him- or herself, verify the patient's identification with a staff member who knows the patient for the second source.	This is another way to double-check identity. Do not use the name on the door or over the bed, because these signs may be inaccurate.
15. Close the door to the room or pull the bedside curtain.	This provides patient privacy.
16. Complete necessary assessments before administering medications. Check the patient's allergy bracelet or ask the patient about allergies. Explain the purpose and action of the medication to the patient.	Assessment is a prerequisite to administration of medications. Explanation provides rationale, increases knowledge, and reduces anxiety.
17. Scan the patient's bar code on the identification band, if required.	Scanning provides an additional check to ensure that the medication is given to the right patient.
18. Assess the IV site for the presence of inflammation or infiltration.	IV medication must be given directly into a vein for safe administration.
19. Close the clamp on the short secondary infusion tubing. Using aseptic technique, remove the cap on the tubing spike and the cap on the port of the medication container, taking care to avoid contaminating either end.	Closing the clamp prevents fluid from entering system until the nurse is ready. Maintaining sterility of the tubing and the medication port prevents contamination.
20. Attach infusion tubing to the medication container by inserting the tubing spike into the port with a firm push and twisting motion, taking care to avoid contaminating either end.	Maintaining sterility of tubing and medication port prevents contamination.

(continued)

Skill · 11   Administering a Piggyback Intermittent Intravenous Infusion of Medication *continued*

ACTION

21. Hang piggyback container on IV pole, positioning it higher than primary IV according to manufacturer's recommendations (Figure 1). Use metal or plastic hook to lower primary IV fluid container. (See the accompanying Skill Variation for information on administering an intermittent IV medication using a tandem piggyback setup.)

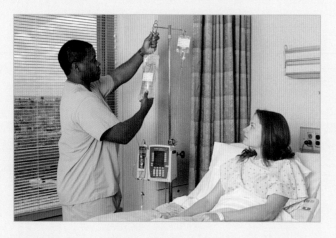

FIGURE 1. Positioning piggyback container on IV pole.

22. Place label on tubing with appropriate date.

23. Squeeze drip chamber on tubing and release. Fill to the line or about half full. Open clamp and prime tubing. Close clamp. Place needleless connector on the end of the tubing, using sterile technique, if required.

24. Use an antimicrobial swab to clean the access port or stopcock above the roller clamp on the primary IV infusion tubing (Figure 2).

25. Connect piggyback setup to the access port or stopcock (Figure 3). If using, turn the stopcock to the open position.

RATIONALE

Position of containers influences the flow of IV fluid into primary setup.

Tubing for piggyback setup may be used for 48 to 96 hours, depending on agency policy. Label allows for tracking of the next date to change.

This removes air from tubing and preserves sterility of setup.

This deters entry of microorganisms when piggyback setup is connected to port. Backflow valve in primary line secondary port stops flow of primary infusion while piggyback solution is infusing. Once completed, backflow valves open and flow of primary solution resumes.

Needleless systems and stopcock setup eliminate the need for a needle and are recommended by the CDC.

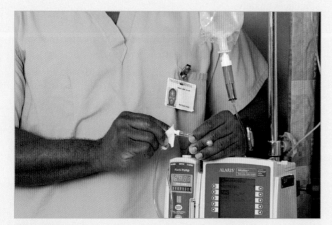

FIGURE 2. Cleaning access port.

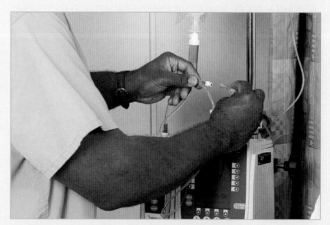

FIGURE 3. Connecting piggyback setup to access port.

ACTION	RATIONALE
26. Open clamp on the secondary tubing. Set rate for secondary infusion on infusion pump and begin infusion (Figure 4). If using gravity infusion, use the roller clamp on the primary infusion tubing to regulate flow at prescribed delivery rate (Figure 5). Monitor medication infusion at periodic intervals.	Backflow valve in primary line secondary port stops flow of primary infusion while piggyback solution is infusing. Once completed, backflow valves open and flow of primary solution resumes. It is important to verify the safe administration rate for each drug to prevent effects.

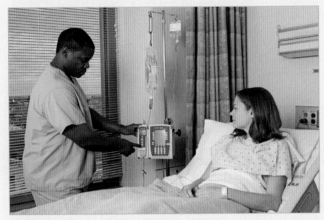

FIGURE 4. Setting rate on infusion pump.

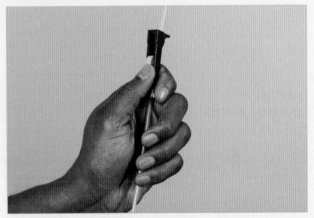

FIGURE 5. Using roller clamp on primary infusion tubing to regulate gravity flow. *(Photo by B. Proud.)*

27. Clamp tubing on piggyback set when solution is infused. Follow facility policy regarding disposal of equipment.	Most facilities allow the reuse of tubing for 48 to 96 hours. This reduces risk for contaminating primary IV setup.
28. Replace primary IV fluid container to original height. **Check primary infusion rate on infusion pump. If using gravity infusion, readjust flow rate of primary IV.**	Most infusion pumps automatically restart primary infusion at previous rate after secondary infusion is completed. If using gravity infusion, piggyback medication administration may interrupt normal flow rate of primary IV. Rate readjustment may be necessary.
29. Remove PPE, if used. Perform hand hygiene.	Removing PPE properly reduces the risk for infection transmission and contamination of other items. Hand hygiene prevents the spread of microorganisms.
30. Document the administration of the medication immediately after administration. See Documentation section below.	Timely documentation helps to ensure patient safety.
31. Evaluate the patient's response to medication within appropriate time frame. Monitor IV site at periodic intervals.	The patient needs to be evaluated for therapeutic and adverse effects from the medication.

EVALUATION

The expected outcomes are met when the medication is delivered via the intravenous route using sterile technique; the medication is delivered to the patient in a safe manner and at the appropriate infusion rate; patient experiences no allergy response; patient remains infection free; and the patient understands and complies with the medication regimen.

DOCUMENTATION

Guidelines

Document the administration of the medication immediately after administration, including date, time, dose, route of administration, site of administration, and rate of administration on the CMAR/MAR or record using the required format. If using a bar-code system, medication administration is automatically recorded when the bar code is scanned. PRN medications require documentation of the reason for administration. Prompt recording avoids the possibility of accidentally repeating the administration of the drug. If the drug was refused or omitted, record this in the appropriate area on the medication record and notify the primary care provider. This verifies the reason medication was omitted and ensures that the primary care provider is aware of the patient's condition. Document the volume of fluid administered on the intake and output record, if necessary.

(continued)

Skill · 11 Administering a Piggyback Intermittent Intravenous Infusion of Medication *continued*

UNEXPECTED SITUATIONS AND ASSOCIATED INTERVENTIONS

- *Upon assessing the IV site before administering medication, you note that the IV has infiltrated:* Stop IV fluid and remove the IV from the extremity. Restart the IV in a different location. Continue to monitor the new IV site as medication is administered.
- *While administering medication, you note a cloudy, white substance forming in the IV tubing:* Stop the IV from flowing and stop administering the medication to prevent precipitate from entering the patient's circulation. Clamp the IV at the site nearest to the patient. Replace tubing on primary and secondary infusions. Check the literature regarding incompatibilities of medications before administering. Medication infusion may require second IV site or flushing of tubing before and after administration, using tandem system.
- *While you are administering medication, the patient begins to complain of pain at the IV site:* Stop the medication. Assess the IV site for any signs of infiltration or phlebitis. Flush the IV with normal saline to check for patency. If the IV site appears within normal limits, resume medication administration at a slower rate.

SPECIAL CONSIDERATIONS

General Considerations

- An alternate way to prime the secondary tubing, particularly if administration set is in place from previous infusion, is to "backfill" the secondary tubing. Attach the medication bag to the secondary infusion tubing. Lower the medication bag below the main IV solution container and open the clamp on the secondary infusion tubing. This allows the primary IV solution to flow up the secondary tubing to the drip chamber, "backfilling" the tubing. Allow the solution to enter the drip chamber until the drip chamber is half full. Close the clamp on the secondary tubing and hang the medication container on the IV pole. Proceed with administration by lowering the primary IV container, as described above. This "backfill" method keeps the infusion system intact, preventing introduction of microorganisms and prevents loss of medication when the tubing is primed. Check facility policy regarding the use of "backfilling."
- Ongoing assessment is an important part of nursing care for both evaluation of patient response to administered medications and early detection of adverse effects. If an adverse effect is suspected, withhold further medication doses and notify the patient's primary healthcare provider. Additional intervention is based on type of reaction and patient assessment.

Infant and Child Considerations

- Small infants and children with fluid restrictions may not tolerate the added IV fluid needed for administration with piggyback or volume-control systems. For these children, consider using the mini-infusion pump.

Skill Variation Tandem Piggyback Setup

A tandem delivery setup allows for simultaneous infusion of the primary and secondary IV solutions. Both solution containers are hung at the same height. The tubing for the secondary infusion is attached to an access port below the roller clamp on the primary tubing. There is no back-check valve at the secondary port on the primary line. This type of setup is used infrequently because the solution from the primary IV line will back up into the tandem line if this intermittent infusion is not clamped immediately after it is infused. It requires a second IV infusion pump to control the rate of the secondary infusion (or the use of primary tubing, if using gravity infusion).

1. Check the medication order against the original order in the medical record, according to facility policy. Clarify any inconsistencies. Check the patient's chart for allergies. Verify the compatibility of the medication and IV fluid.

2. Know the actions, special nursing considerations, safe dose ranges, purpose of administration, and adverse effects of the medications to be administered. Consider the appropriateness of the medication for this patient.

3. Perform hand hygiene.

4. Move the medication cart to the outside of the patient's room or prepare for administration in the medication area.

5. Unlock the medication cart or drawer. Enter pass code and scan employee identification, if required.

6. Read the CMAR/MAR and select the proper medication from the patient's medication drawer or unit stock.

7. Compare the label with the CMAR/MAR. Check the expiration dates. Confirm the prescribed or appropriate infusion rate. Calculate the drip rate if using gravity system. Scan the bar code on the package, if required.

8. **Recheck the label with the CMAR/MAR before taking it to the patient.** Some facilities require the third check to occur at the bedside, after identifying the patient and before administration.

Skill Variation   Tandem Piggyback Setup   *continued*

9. Lock the medication cart before leaving it.

10. Transport medications and equipment to the patient's bedside carefully, and keep the medications in sight at all times.

11. **Ensure that the patient receives the medications at the correct time.**

12. Perform hand hygiene and put on PPE, if indicated.

13. Identify the patient. The patient should be identified using two methods.

14. Close the door to the room or pull the bedside curtain.

15. Complete necessary assessments before administering medications. Check the patient's allergy bracelet or ask the patient about allergies. Explain the purpose and action of the medication to the patient.

16. Scan the patient's bar code on the identification band, if required.

17. Assess the IV site for the presence of inflammation or infiltration.

18. Close the clamp on the secondary infusion tubing. Using aseptic technique, remove the cap on the tubing spike and the cap on the port of the medication container, taking care not to contaminate either end.

19. Attach infusion tubing to the medication container by inserting the tubing spike into the port with a firm push and twisting motion, taking care not to contaminate either end.

20. Hang secondary container on IV pole, positioning it at the same height as the primary IV.

21. Place label on tubing with appropriate date.

22. Squeeze drip chamber and release. Fill to the line or about half full. Open clamp and prime tubing. Close clamp. Place needleless connector on the end of the tubing using sterile technique, if required. Insert tubing into infusion pump, according to manufacturer's directions.

23. Use an antimicrobial swab to clean the access port or stopcock below the roller clamp on the primary IV infusion tubing, usually the port closest to the IV insertion site.

24. Connect secondary setup to the access port or stopcock. If using, turn the stopcock to the open position.

25. Open clamp on the secondary tubing. Set rate for secondary infusion on infusion pump. If using gravity infusion, use the roller clamp on the primary infusion tubing to regulate flow at prescribed delivery rate. Monitor medication infusion at periodic intervals.

26. Turn off secondary infusion pump. Clamp tubing on secondary set when solution is infused. Remove secondary tubing from access port and cap, or replace connector with a new, capped one, if reusing. Follow facility policy regarding disposal of equipment.

27. Check primary infusion rate.

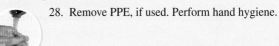

28. Remove PPE, if used. Perform hand hygiene.

29. Evaluate the patient's response to medication within appropriate time frame. Monitor IV site at periodic intervals.

EVIDENCE FOR PRACTICE

"Smart Pumps"

Medication errors occur frequently and are a serious problem in healthcare. Medication errors may have serious consequences. Healthcare institutions and healthcare providers have a responsibility to prevent medication errors. "Smart pump" technology is one intervention to use to reduce medication errors.

Related Research

Rosenkoetter, M., Bowcutt, M., Khasanshina, E., et al. (2008). Perceptions of the impact of "Smart Pumps" on nurses and nursing care provided. *Journal of the Association for Vascular Access, 13*(2), 60–69.

This study focused on the perceptions of nurses regarding the impact of the implementation of "smart pump" technology and on nursing care provided, medication errors, and job satisfaction. Results indicate that the nurses perceived that the use of the pumps increased safe medication administration, did not decrease the perception of the punitive nature of reporting medication errors, and did not increase the nurses' workload. The participants also reported that the use of the pumps made daily routines easier. The pump was perceived to increase self-confidence but had no effect on the use of pharmacy staff. The pump also increased patient/family confidence in care received. There was no relationship with age, years of nursing experience, and staff nursing degree earned.

Relevance to Nursing Practice

Nurses should welcome the adoption of new technologies to improve nursing practice and decrease medication errors. This study reinforces that technology is easy to use and should not be feared; the use of smart pumps can increase both job satisfaction and self-confidence and decrease anxiety of making IV medication errors. The importance of the perceptions of the nursing staff in the implementation of new technology should be considered by a facility that is planning a major technological change.

Skill · 12   Administering an Intermittent Intravenous Infusion of Medication via a Mini-infusion Pump

With intermittent IV infusion, the drug is mixed with a small amount of the IV solution, and administered over a short period at the prescribed interval (e.g., every 4 hours). The mini-infusion pump (syringe pump) for intermittent infusion is battery or electrical operated and allows medication mixed in a syringe to be connected to the primary line and delivered by mechanical pressure applied to the syringe plunger (Figure 1). "Smart (computerized) pumps" are being used by many facilities for IV infusions, including intermittent infusions. Smart pumps also require programming of infusion rates by the nurse, but also are able to identify dosing limits and practice guidelines to aid in safe administration.

EQUIPMENT

- Medication prepared in labeled syringe
- Mini-infusion pump and tubing
- Needleless connector, if required, based on facility system
- Antimicrobial swab
- Date label for tubing
- Computer-generated Medication Administration Record (CMAR) or Medication Administration Record (MAR)
- PPE, as indicated

ASSESSMENT

Assess the patient for any allergies. Check the expiration date before administering medication. Assess the appropriateness of the drug for the patient. Assess the compatibility of the ordered medication, diluent, and the infusing IV fluid. Review assessment and laboratory data that may influence drug administration. Verify patient name, dose, route, and time of administration. Assess the patient's knowledge of the medication. If the patient has a knowledge deficit about the medication, this may be the appropriate time to begin education about the medication. If the medication may affect the patient's vital signs, assess them before administration. Assess the IV insertion site, noting any swelling, coolness, leakage of fluid at site, redness, or pain.

NURSING DIAGNOSIS

Determine related factors for the nursing diagnoses based on the patient's current status. Appropriate nursing diagnoses include:

- Risk for Allergy Response
- Deficient Knowledge
- Risk for Injury
- Risk for Infection

OUTCOME IDENTIFICATION AND PLANNING

The expected outcome is that the medication is delivered via the intravenous route using sterile technique. Other outcomes that may be appropriate include the following: medication is delivered to the patient in a safe manner and at the appropriate infusion rate; patient experiences no allergy response; patient remains infection free; and the patient understands and complies with the medication regimen.

IMPLEMENTATION

ACTION	RATIONALE
1. Gather equipment. Check each medication order against the original order in the medical record according to facility policy. Clarify any inconsistencies. Check the patient's chart for allergies.	This comparison helps to identify errors that may have occurred when orders were transcribed. The primary care provider order is the legal record of medication orders for each facility.
2. Know the actions, special nursing considerations, safe dose ranges, purpose of administration, and adverse effects of the medications to be administered. Consider the appropriateness of the medication for this patient.	This knowledge aids the nurse in evaluating the therapeutic effect of the medication in relation to the patient's disorder and can also be used to educate the patient about the medication.
3. Perform hand hygiene.	Hand hygiene prevents the spread of microorganisms.
4. Move the medication cart to the outside of the patient's room or prepare for administration in the medication area.	Organization facilitates error-free administration and saves time.

ACTION	RATIONALE
5. Unlock the medication cart or drawer. Enter pass code and scan employee identification, if required.	Locking the cart or drawer safeguards each patient's medication supply. Hospital accrediting organizations require medication carts to be locked when not in use. Entering pass code and scanning ID allows only authorized users into the system and identifies user for documentation by the computer.
6. **Prepare medications for one patient at a time.**	This prevents errors in medication administration.
7. Read the CMAR/MAR and select the proper medication from the patient's medication drawer or unit stock.	This is the *first* check of the label.
8. Compare the label with the CMAR/MAR. Check expiration dates. Confirm the prescribed or appropriate infusion rate. Scan the bar code on the package, if required.	This is the *second* check of the label. Verify calculations with another nurse to ensure safety, if necessary. Infusing medication at appropriate rate prevents injury.
9. **When all medications for one patient have been prepared, recheck the label with the MAR before taking them to the patient.**	This is the *third* check to ensure accuracy and to prevent errors. Some facilities require the third check to occur at the bedside, after identifying the patient and before administration.
10. Lock the medication cart before leaving it.	Locking the cart or drawer safeguards the patient's medication supply. Hospital accrediting organizations require medication carts to be locked when not in use.
11. Transport medications to the patient's bedside carefully, and keep the medications in sight at all times.	Careful handling and close observation prevent accidental or deliberate disarrangement of medications.
12. **Ensure that the patient receives the medications at the correct time.**	Check facility policy, which may allow for administration within a period of 30 minutes before or 30 minutes after designated time.
13. Perform hand hygiene and put on PPE, if indicated.	Hand hygiene and PPE prevent the spread of microorganisms. PPE is required based on transmission precautions.
14. Identify the patient. Usually, the patient should be identified using two methods. Compare information with the MAR/CMAR.	Identifying the patient ensures the right patient receives the medications and helps prevent errors.
a. Check the name and identification number on the patient's identification band.	This is the most reliable method. Replace the identification band if it is missing or inaccurate in any way.
b. Ask the patient to state his or her name and birth date, based on facility policy.	This requires a response from the patient, but illness and strange surroundings often cause patients to be confused.
c. If the patient cannot identify him- or herself, verify the patient's identification with a staff member who knows the patient for the second source.	This is another way to double-check identity. Do not use the name on the door or over the bed, because these signs may be inaccurate.
15. Close the door to the room or pull the bedside curtain.	Provides patient privacy.
16. Complete necessary assessments before administering medications. Check the patient's allergy bracelet or ask the patient about allergies. Explain the purpose and action of the medication to the patient.	Assessment is a prerequisite to administration of medications. Explanation provides rationale, increases knowledge, and reduces anxiety.
17. Scan the patient's bar code on the identification band, if required.	Provides an additional check to ensure that the medication is given to the right patient.
18. Assess the IV site for the presence of inflammation or infiltration.	IV medication must be given directly into a vein for safe administration.
19. Using aseptic technique, remove the cap on the tubing and the cap on the syringe, taking care not to contaminate either end.	Maintaining sterility of tubing and syringe prevents contamination.
20. Attach infusion tubing to the syringe, taking care not to contaminate either end.	Maintaining sterility of tubing and medication port prevents contamination.

(continued)

Skill · 12   **Administering an Intermittent Intravenous Infusion of Medication via a Mini-infusion Pump** *continued*

ACTION	RATIONALE
21. Place label on tubing with appropriate date.	Tubing for piggyback setup may be used for 48 to 96 hours, depending on facility policy. Label allows for tracking of the next date to change.
22. Fill tubing with medication by applying gentle pressure to syringe plunger. Place needleless connector on the end of the tubing, using sterile technique, if required.	This removes air from tubing and maintains sterility.
23. Insert syringe into mini-infusion pump according to manufacturer's directions (Figure 1).	Syringe must fit securely in pump apparatus for proper operation.
24. Use antimicrobial swab to clean the access port or stopcock below the roller clamp on the primary IV infusion tubing, usually the port closest to the IV insertion site (Figure 2).	This deters entry of microorganisms when the piggyback setup is connected to the port. Proper connection allows IV medication to flow into primary line.

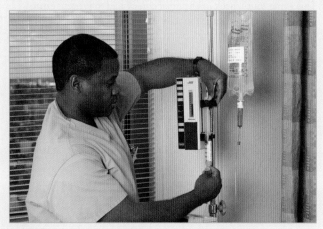

FIGURE 1. Inserting syringe into mini-infusion pump.

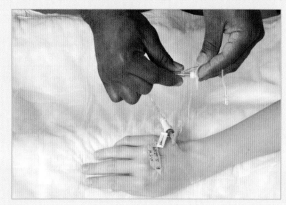

FIGURE 2. Cleaning access port closest to IV insertion site.

25. Connect the secondary infusion to the primary infusion at the cleansed port (Figure 3).	Allows for delivery of medication.
26. Program pump to the appropriate rate and begin infusion (Figure 4). Set alarm if recommended by manufacturer.	Pump delivers medication at a controlled rate. Alarm is recommended for use with IV lock apparatus.

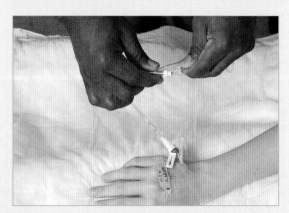

FIGURE 3. Connecting secondary infusion tubing to primary infusion.

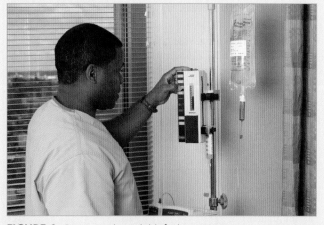

FIGURE 4. Programming mini-infusion pump.

27. Clamp tubing on secondary set when solution is infused. Remove secondary tubing from access port and cap, or replace connector with a new, capped one, if reusing. Follow facility policy regarding disposal of equipment.	Many facilities allow reuse of tubing for 48 to 96 hours. Replacing connector or needle with a new, capped one maintains system sterility.

ACTION	RATIONALE
28. Check rate of primary infusion.	Administration of secondary infusion may interfere with primary infusion rate.
29. Remove PPE, if used. Perform hand hygiene.	Removing PPE properly reduces the risk for infection transmission and contamination of other items. Hand hygiene prevents the spread of microorganisms.
30. Document the administration of the medication immediately after administration. See Documentation section below.	Timely documentation helps to ensure patient safety.
31. Evaluate the patient's response to medication within appropriate time frame. Monitor IV site at periodic intervals.	The patient needs to be evaluated for therapeutic and adverse effects from the medication.

EVALUATION

The expected outcomes are met when the medication is delivered via the intravenous route using sterile technique; the medication is delivered to the patient in a safe manner and at the appropriate infusion rate; patient experiences no allergy response; patient remains infection free; and the patient understands and complies with the medication regimen.

DOCUMENTATION
Guidelines

Document the administration of the medication immediately after administration, including date, time, dose, route of administration, site of administration, and rate of administration on the CMAR/MAR or record using the required format. If using a bar-code system, medication administration is automatically recorded when bar code is scanned. PRN medications require documentation of the reason for administration. Prompt recording avoids the possibility of accidentally repeating the administration of the drug. If the drug was refused or omitted, record this in the appropriate area on the medication record and notify the primary care provider. This verifies the reason medication was omitted and ensures that the primary care provider is aware of the patient's condition. Document the volume of fluid administered on the intake and output record, if necessary.

UNEXPECTED SITUATIONS AND ASSOCIATED INTERVENTIONS

- *Upon assessing the IV site before administering medication, you note that the IV has infiltrated:* Stop IV fluid and remove the IV from the extremity. Restart the IV in a different location. Continue to monitor the new IV site as medication is administered.
- *While administering medication, you note a cloudy, white substance forming in the IV tubing:* Stop the IV from flowing and stop administering the medication to prevent precipitate from entering the patient's circulation. Clamp the IV at the site nearest to the patient. Replace tubing on primary and secondary infusions. Check the literature regarding incompatibilities of medications before administering. Medication infusion may require a second IV site or flushing of tubing before and after administration.
- *While you are administering medication, the patient begins to complain of pain at the IV site:* Stop the medication. Assess the IV site for any signs of infiltration or phlebitis. Flush the IV with normal saline to check for patency. If the IV site appears within normal limits, resume medication administration at a slower rate.

SPECIAL CONSIDERATIONS

- Ongoing assessment is an important part of nursing care for both evaluation of patient response to administered medications and early detection of adverse effects. If an adverse effect is suspected, withhold further medication doses and notify the patient's primary healthcare provider. Additional intervention is based on type of reaction and patient assessment.

EVIDENCE FOR PRACTICE

"Smart Pumps"
Medication errors occur frequently and are a serious problem in healthcare. Medication errors may have serious consequences. Healthcare institutions and healthcare providers have a responsibility to prevent medication errors. "Smart pump" technology is one intervention to use to reduce errors.
Refer to the Evidence for Practice feature at the end of Skill 5-11 for related research.

Skill · 13   Administering an Intermittent Intravenous Infusion of Medication via a Volume-Control Administration Set

With intermittent IV infusion, the drug is mixed with a small amount of the IV solution, such as 50 to 100 mL, and administered over a short period at the prescribed interval (e.g., every 4 hours). The administration is most often performed using an IV infusion pump, which requires the nurse to program the infusion rate into the pump. "Smart (computerized) pumps" are being used by many facilities for IV infusions, including intermittent infusions. Smart pumps also require programming of infusion rates by the nurse, but also are able to identify dosing limits and practice guidelines to aid in safe administration. Administration may be achieved by gravity infusion, which requires the nurse to calculate the infusion rate in drops per minute. The best practice, however, is to use an intravenous infusion pump.

This skill discusses using a volume-control administration set for intermittent IV infusion. The medication is diluted with a small amount of solution and administered through the patient's IV line. This type of equipment is commonly used for infusing solutions into children, critically ill patients, and older patients when the volume of fluid infused is a concern. Needleless devices (recommended by the CDC and the Occupational Safety and Health Administration [OSHA]) prevent needlesticks and provide access to the primary venous line. Either a blunt-ended cannula or a recessed connection port may be used to connect intermittent IV infusions.

EQUIPMENT

- Prescribed medication
- Syringe with a needless device or blunt needle, if required, based on facility system
- Volume-control set (Volutrol, Buretrol, Burette)
- Needleless connector or stopcock, if required
- Infusion pump, if needed
- Antimicrobial swab
- Date label for tubing
- Medication label
- Computer-generated Medication Administration Record (CMAR) or Medication Administration Record (MAR)
- PPE, as indicated

ASSESSMENT

Assess the patient for any allergies. Check the expiration date before administering medication. Assess the appropriateness of the drug for the patient. Assess the compatibility of the ordered medication, diluent, and the infusing IV fluid. Review assessment and laboratory data that may influence drug administration. Assess the patient's knowledge of the medication. If the patient has a knowledge deficit about the medication, this may be the appropriate time to begin education about the medication. If the medication may affect the patient's vital signs, assess them before administration. Assess the IV insertion site, noting any swelling, coolness, leakage of fluid at site, redness, or pain.

NURSING DIAGNOSIS

Determine related factors for the nursing diagnoses based on the patient's current status. Appropriate nursing diagnoses include:

- Risk for Allergy Response
- Deficient Knowledge
- Risk for Injury
- Risk for Infection

OUTCOME IDENTIFICATION AND PLANNING

The expected outcome to achieve when administering an intermittent IV infusion of medication via a volume control set is that the medication is delivered via the intravenous route using sterile technique. Other outcomes that may be appropriate include the following: medication is delivered to the patient in a safe manner and at the appropriate infusion rate; patient experiences no allergy response; patient remains infection free; and the patient understands and complies with the medication regimen.

IMPLEMENTATION

ACTION	RATIONALE
1. Gather equipment. Check the medication order against the original order in the medical record according to facility policy. Clarify any inconsistencies. Check the patient's chart for allergies. Verify the compatibility of the medication and IV fluid.	This comparison helps to identify errors that may have occurred when orders were transcribed. The primary care provider's order is the legal record of medication orders for each facility. Compatibility of medication and solution prevents complications.

ACTION

RATIONALE

2. Know the actions, special nursing considerations, safe dose ranges, purpose of administration, and adverse effects of the medications to be administered. Consider the appropriateness of the medication for this patient.

This knowledge aids the nurse in evaluating the therapeutic effect of the medication in relation to the patient's disorder and can also be used to educate the patient about the medication.

3. Perform hand hygiene.

Hand hygiene prevents the spread of microorganisms.

4. Move the medication cart to the outside of the patient's room or prepare for administration in the medication area.

Organization facilitates error-free administration and saves time.

5. Unlock the medication cart or drawer. Enter pass code and scan employee identification, if required.

Locking of the cart or drawer safeguards each patient's medication supply. Hospital accrediting organizations require medication carts to be locked when not in use. Entering pass code and scanning ID allows only authorized users into the system and identifies user for documentation by the computer.

6. **Prepare medication for one patient at a time.**

This prevents errors in medication administration.

7. Read the CMAR/MAR and select the proper medication from the patient's medication drawer or unit stock.

This is the *first* check of the label.

8. Compare the label with the CMAR/MAR. Check expiration dates and perform calculations, if necessary. Confirm the prescribed or appropriate infusion rate. Calculate the drip rate if using gravity system. Scan the bar code on the package, if required. Check the infusion rate.

This is the *second* check of the label. Verify calculations with another nurse to ensure safety, if necessary. Delivers the correct dose of medication as prescribed.

9. If necessary, withdraw medication from an ampule or vial as described in Skills 5-3 and 5-4. Attach needleless connector or blunt needle to end of syringe, if necessary.

Allows for entry into the volume-control administration set chamber.

10. **When all medications for one patient have been prepared, recheck the label with the CMAR/MAR before taking them to the patient.**

This is the *third* check to ensure accuracy and to prevent errors. Some facilities require the third check to occur at the bedside, after identifying the patient and before administration.

11. Prepare medication label including name of medication, dose, total volume, including diluent, and time of administration.

Allows for accurate identification of medication.

12. Lock the medication cart before leaving it.

Locking the cart or drawer safeguards the patient's medication supply. Hospital accrediting organizations require medication carts to be locked when not in use.

13. Transport medications and equipment to the patient's bedside carefully, and keep the medications in sight at all times.

Careful handling and close observation prevent accidental or deliberate disarrangement of medications. Having equipment available saves time and facilitates performance of the task.

14. **Ensure that the patient receives the medications at the correct time.**

Check facility policy, which may allow for administration within a period of 30 minutes before or 30 minutes after designated time.

15. Perform hand hygiene and put on PPE, if indicated.

Hand hygiene and PPE prevent the spread of microorganisms. PPE is required based on transmission precautions.

16. Identify the patient. Usually, the patient should be identified using two methods. Compare information with the CMAR/MAR.

Identifying the patient ensures the right patient receives the medications and helps prevent errors.

a. Check the name and identification number on the patient's identification band.

This is the most reliable method. Replace the identification band if it is missing or inaccurate in any way.

(continued)

Skill · 13 Administering an Intermittent Intravenous Infusion of Medication via a Volume-Control Administration Set *continued*

ACTION	RATIONALE
b. Ask the patient to state his or her name and birth date, based on facility policy.	This requires a response from the patient, but illness and strange surroundings often cause patients to be confused.
c. If the patient cannot identify him- or herself, verify the patient's identification with a staff member who knows the patient for the second source.	This is another way to double-check identity. Do not use the name on the door or over the bed, because these signs may be inaccurate.
17. Close the door to the room or pull the bedside curtain.	This provides patient privacy.
18. Complete necessary assessments before administering medications. Check the patient's allergy bracelet or ask the patient about allergies. Explain the purpose and action of the medication to the patient.	Assessment is a prerequisite to administration of medications. Explanation provides rationale, increases knowledge, and reduces anxiety.
19. Scan the patient's bar code on the identification band, if required.	Provides an additional check to ensure that the medication is given to the right patient.
20. Assess IV site for presence of inflammation or infiltration.	IV medication must be given directly into a vein for safe administration.
21. Fill the volume-control administration set (Figure 1) with the prescribed amount of IV fluid by opening the clamp between IV solution and the volume-control administration set. Follow manufacturer's instructions and fill with prescribed amount of IV solution (Figure 2). Close clamp.	This dilutes the medication in the minimal amount of solution. Reclamping prevents the continued addition of fluid to the volume to be mixed with medication.
22. Check to make sure the air vent on the volume-control administration set chamber is open.	Air vent allows fluid in the chamber to flow at a regular rate.
23. Use antimicrobial swab to clean access port on volume-control administration set chamber (Figure 3).	This deters entry of microorganisms when the syringe enters the chamber.

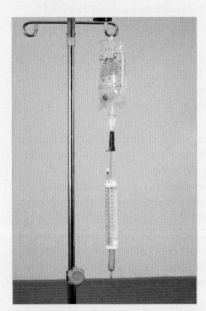

FIGURE 1. Volume-control administration set and IV solution for dilution of medication. *(Photo by B. Proud.)*

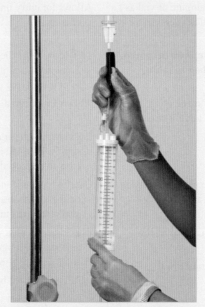

FIGURE 2. Opening clamp between IV solution and volume-control administration set to fill chamber with prescribed amount of solution. *(Photo by B. Proud.)*

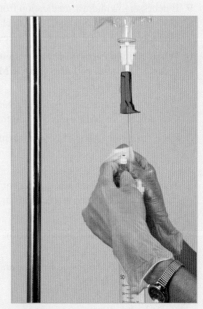

FIGURE 3. Cleaning access port. *(Photo by B. Proud.)*

24. Attach the syringe with a twisting motion into the access port while holding the syringe steady (Figure 4). Alternately, insert the needleless device or blunt needle into the port. Inject the medication into the chamber (Figure 5). Gently rotate the chamber.	This ensures that medication is evenly mixed with the solution.

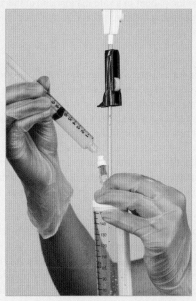

FIGURE 4. Attaching syringe to access port. *(Photo by B. Proud.)*

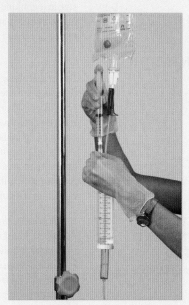

FIGURE 5. Adding medication to the chamber. *(Photo by B. Proud.)*

25. Attach the medication label to the volume-control device.

This identifies contents of the set and prevents medication error.

26. Use an antimicrobial swab to clean the access port or stopcock below the roller clamp on the primary IV infusion tubing, usually the port closest to the IV insertion site.

This deters entry of microorganisms when the piggyback setup is connected to the port. Proper connection allows IV medication to flow into primary line.

27. Connect the secondary infusion to the primary infusion at the cleansed port.

This allows for delivery of medication.

28. The volume-control administration set may be placed on an infusion pump with the appropriate dose programmed into the pump. Alternately, use the roller clamp on the volume-control administration set tubing to adjust the infusion to the prescribed rate.

Delivery over a 30- to 60-minute interval is a safe method of administering IV medication.

29. Discard the syringe in the appropriate receptacle.

Proper disposal prevents injury.

30. Clamp tubing on secondary set when solution is infused. Remove secondary tubing from access port and cap or replace connector with a new, capped one, if reusing. Follow facility policy regarding disposal of equipment.

Many facilities allow reuse of tubing for 48 to 96 hours. Replacing connector or needle with a new, capped one maintains sterility of system.

31. Check rate of primary infusion.

Administration of secondary infusion may interfere with primary infusion rate.

 32. Remove PPE, if used. Perform hand hygiene.

Removing PPE properly reduces the risk for infection transmission and contamination of other items. Hand hygiene prevents the spread of microorganisms.

33. Document the administration of the medication immediately after administration. See Documentation section below.

Timely documentation helps to ensure patient safety.

34. Evaluate the patient's response to medication within appropriate time frame. Monitor IV site at periodic intervals.

The patient needs to be evaluated for therapeutic and adverse effects from the medication. Visualization of the site also allows for assessment of any untoward effects.

(continued)

Skill · 13   Administering an Intermittent Intravenous Infusion of Medication via a Volume-Control Administration Set   *continued*

EVALUATION

The expected outcomes are met when the medication is delivered via the intravenous route using sterile technique; the medication is delivered to the patient in a safe manner and at the appropriate infusion rate; patient experiences no allergy response; patient remains infection free; and the patient understands and complies with the medication regimen.

DOCUMENTATION
Guidelines

Document the administration of the medication immediately after administration, including date, time, dose, route of administration, site of administration, and rate of administration on the CMAR/MAR or record using the required format. If using a bar-code system, medication administration is automatically recorded when the bar code is scanned. PRN medications require documentation of the reason for administration. Prompt recording avoids the possibility of accidentally repeating the administration of the drug. If the drug was refused or omitted, record this in the appropriate area on the medication record and notify the primary care provider. This verifies the reason medication was omitted and ensures that the primary care provider is aware of the patient's condition. Document the volume of fluid administered on the intake and output record, if necessary.

UNEXPECTED SITUATIONS AND ASSOCIATED INTERVENTIONS

- *Upon assessing the IV site before administering medication, you note that the IV has infiltrated:* Stop IV fluid and remove the IV from the extremity. Restart the IV in a different location. Continue to monitor the new IV site as medication is administered.
- *While administering medication, you note a cloudy, white substance forming in the IV tubing:* Stop the IV from flowing and stop administering the medication to prevent precipitate from entering the patient's circulation. Clamp the IV at the site nearest to the patient. Replace tubing on primary and secondary infusions. Check the literature regarding incompatibilities of medications before administering. Medication infusion may require second IV site or flushing of tubing before and after administration.
- *While you are administering medication, the patient begins to complain of pain at the IV site:* Stop the medication. Assess the IV site for any signs of infiltration or phlebitis. Flush the IV with normal saline to check for patency. If the IV site appears within normal limits, resume medication administration at a slower rate.

SPECIAL CONSIDERATIONS

- Ongoing assessment is an important part of nursing care to evaluate patient response to administered medications and early detection of adverse effects. If an adverse effect is suspected, withhold further medication doses and notify the patient's primary healthcare provider. Additional intervention is based on type of reaction and patient assessment.

EVIDENCE FOR PRACTICE

"Smart Pumps"
Medication errors occur frequently and are a serious problem in healthcare. Medication errors may have serious consequences. Healthcare institutions and healthcare providers have a responsibility to prevent medication errors. "Smart pump" technology is one intervention to use to reduce errors.
Refer to the Evidence for Practice feature at the end of Skill 5-11 for related research.

Skill · 14   Introducing Drugs Through a Medication or Drug-Infusion Lock (Intermittent Peripheral Venous Access Device) Using the Saline Flush

A medication or drug-infusion lock, also known as an intermittent peripheral venous access device, is used for patients who require intermittent IV medication, but not a continuous IV infusion. This device consists of a needle or catheter connected to a short length of tubing capped with a sealed injection port. After the catheter is in place in the patient's vein, the catheter and tubing are anchored to the patient's arm so that the catheter remains in place until the patient no longer requires the repeated medication intravenously.

A peripheral venous access device allows the patient more freedom than a continuous IV infusion. The patient is connected to the IV line when it is time to receive the medication and disconnected when the medication is completed. The device is kept patent (working) by flushing with small amounts of saline pushed through the device on a routine basis. Using saline eliminates any possible systemic effects on coagulation, development of a heparin allergy, and drug incompatibility, which may occur when a heparin solution is used. The intermittent infusion is not started until the nurse confirms IV placement. The saline lock is flushed before the infusion is begun and after the infusion is completed to clear the vein of any medication and to prevent clot formation in the needle. If infiltration or phlebitis occurs, the lock is removed and replaced in a new site.

EQUIPMENT

- Medication
- Saline flushes (2), volume according to facility policy, usually 2 to 3 mL
- Antimicrobial swabs
- Watch with second hand or stopwatch feature
- Gloves
- Computer-generated Medication Administration Record (CMAR) or Medication Administration Record (MAR)

ASSESSMENT

Assess the patient for any allergies. Check the expiration date before administering medication. Assess the appropriateness of the drug for the patient. Assess the compatibility of the ordered medication and the IV fluid. Review assessment and laboratory data that may influence drug administration. Assess patient's IV site, noting any swelling, coolness, leakage of fluid from IV site, or pain. Assess the patient's knowledge of the medication. If the patient has a knowledge deficit about the medication, this may be the appropriate time to begin education about the medication. If the medication may affect the patient's vital signs, assess them before administration. If the medication is for pain relief, assess the patient's pain before and after administration.

NURSING DIAGNOSIS

Determine related factors for the nursing diagnoses based on the patient's current status. Appropriate nursing diagnoses may include:
- Risk for Allergy Response
- Risk for Infection
- Risk for Injury
- Deficient Knowledge

OUTCOME IDENTIFICATION AND PLANNING

The expected outcome to achieve when administering an intermittent IV infusion of medication via a medication or drug-infusion lock is that the medication is delivered via the intravenous route using sterile technique. Other outcomes that may be appropriate include the following: medication is delivered to the patient in a safe manner and at the appropriate infusion rate; patient experiences no adverse effect; and the patient understands and complies with the medication regimen.

IMPLEMENTATION

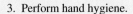

ACTION

1. Gather equipment. Check the medication order against the original order in the medical record, according to agency policy. Clarify any inconsistencies. Check the patient's chart for allergies. Check a drug resource to clarify whether medication needs to be diluted before administration. Verify the recommended infusion rate.

2. Know the actions, special nursing considerations, safe dose ranges, purpose of administration, and adverse effects of the medications to be administered. Consider the appropriateness of the medication for this patient.

   3. Perform hand hygiene.

RATIONALE

This comparison helps to identify errors that may have occurred when orders were transcribed. The physician's order is the legal record of medication orders for each agency. Compatibility of medication and solution prevents complications. Recommended infusion rate delivers the correct dose of medication as prescribed.

This knowledge aids the nurse in evaluating the therapeutic effect of the medication in relation to the patient's disorder and can also be used to educate the patient about the medication.

Hand hygiene prevents the spread of microorganisms.

(continued)

Skill · 14   Introducing Drugs Through a Medication or Drug-Infusion Lock (Intermittent Peripheral Venous Access Device) Using the Saline Flush   *continued*

ACTION	RATIONALE
4. Move the medication cart to the outside of the patient's room or prepare for administration in the medication area.	Organization facilitates error-free administration and saves time.
5. Unlock the medication cart or drawer. Enter pass code and scan employee identification, if required.	Locking the cart or drawer safeguards each patient's medication supply. Hospital accrediting organizations require medication carts to be locked when not in use. Entering pass code and scanning ID allows only authorized users into the system and identifies user for documentation by the computer.
6. **Prepare medication for one patient at a time.**	This prevents errors in medication administration.
7. Read the CMAR/MAR and select the proper medication from the patient's medication drawer or unit stock.	This is the *first* check of the label.
8. Compare the label with the CMAR/MAR. Check expiration dates and perform calculations, if necessary. Scan the bar code on the package, if required.	This is the *second* check of the label. Verify calculations with another nurse to ensure safety, if necessary.
9. If necessary, withdraw medication from an ampule or vial as described in Skills 5-3 and 5-4.	Allows administration of medication.
10. **When all medications for one patient have been prepared, recheck the label with the MAR before taking them to the patient.**	This is the *third* check to ensure accuracy and to prevent errors. Some facilities require the third check to occur at the bedside, after identifying the patient and before administration.
11. Lock the medication cart before leaving it.	Locking the cart or drawer safeguards the patient's medication supply. Hospital accrediting organizations require medication carts to be locked when not in use.
12. Transport medications and equipment to the patient's bedside carefully, and keep the medications in sight at all times.	Careful handling and close observation prevent accidental or deliberate disarrangement of medications. Having equipment available saves time and facilitates performance of the task.
13. **Ensure that the patient receives the medications at the correct time.**	Check facility policy, which may allow for administration within a period of 30 minutes before or 30 minutes after designated time.
14. Perform hand hygiene and put on PPE, if indicated.	Hand hygiene and PPE prevent the spread of microorganisms. PPE is required based on transmission precautions.
15. Identify the patient. Usually, the patient should be identified using two methods. Compare information with the MAR/CMAR.	Identifying the patient ensures the right patient receives the medications and helps prevent errors.
a. Check the name and identification number on the patient's identification band.	This is the most reliable method. Replace the identification band if it is missing or inaccurate in any way.
b. Ask the patient to state his or her name and birth date, based on facility policy.	This requires a response from the patient, but illness and strange surroundings often cause patients to be confused.
c. If the patient cannot identify him- or herself, verify the patient's identification with a staff member who knows the patient for the second source.	This is another way to double-check identity. Do not use the name on the door or over the bed, because these signs may be inaccurate.
16. Close the door to the room or pull the bedside curtain.	This provides patient privacy.
17. Complete necessary assessments before administering medications. Check the patient's allergy bracelet or ask the patient about allergies. Explain the purpose and action of the medication to the patient.	Assessment is a prerequisite to administration of medications. Explanation provides rationale, increases knowledge, and reduces anxiety.
18 Scan the patient's bar code on the identification band, if required.	Scanning provides an additional check to ensure that the medication is given to the right patient.
19. Assess IV site for presence of inflammation or infiltration.	IV medication must be given directly into a vein for safe administration.

ACTION	**RATIONALE**
20. Put on clean gloves.	Gloves protect the nurse's hands from contact with the patient's blood.
21. Clean the access port of the medication lock with antimicrobial swab (Figure 1).	Cleaning removes surface contaminants at the lock entry site.
22. Stabilize the port with your nondominant hand and insert the syringe, or needleless access device, of normal saline into the access port (Figure 2).	This allows for careful insertion into the center circle of the lock.
23. Release the clamp on the extension tubing of the medication lock. Aspirate gently and check for blood return (Figure 3).	This ensures the catheter of the medication lock is in a vein.

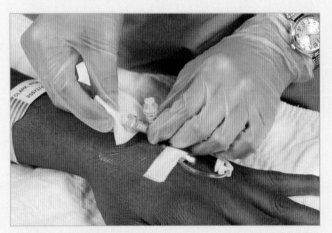

FIGURE 1. Cleaning access port. *(Photo by B. Proud.)*

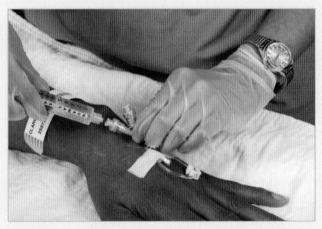

FIGURE 2. Inserting syringe into access port. *(Photo by B. Proud.)*

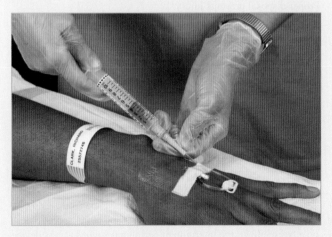

FIGURE 3. Aspirating for blood return. *(Photo by B. Proud.)*

24. Gently flush with normal saline by pushing slowly on the syringe plunger. Observe the insertion site while inserting the saline. Remove syringe.	Saline flush ensures that the IV line is patent. Puffiness or swelling as the site is flushed could indicate infiltration of the catheter.
25. Insert syringe, or needleless access device, with medication into the port and gently inject medication, using a watch to verify correct administration rate. **Do not force the injection if resistance is felt.**	Easy installation of medication usually indicates that the lock is still patent and in the vein. If force is used against resistance, a clot may break away and cause a blockage elsewhere in the body.

(continued)

Skill · 14 | **Introducing Drugs Through a Medication or Drug-Infusion Lock (Intermittent Peripheral Venous Access Device) Using the Saline Flush** *continued*

ACTION

26. Remove the medication syringe from the port. Stabilize the port with your nondominant hand and insert the syringe, or needleless access device, of normal saline into the port. Gently flush with normal saline by pushing slowly on the syringe plunger (Figure 4). **If medication lock is capped with positive pressure valve/device, remove syringe, and then clamp the IV tubing (Figure 5).** Alternately, to gain positive pressure if positive pressure valve/device is not present, clamp the IV tubing as you are still flushing the last of the saline into the medication lock. Remove syringe.

RATIONALE

Positive pressure prevents blood from backing into the catheter and causing the medication lock to clot off.

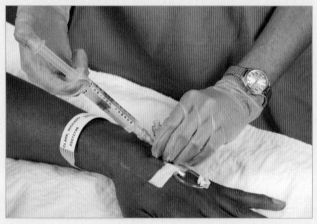

FIGURE 4. Flushing port with normal saline. *(Photo by B. Proud.)*

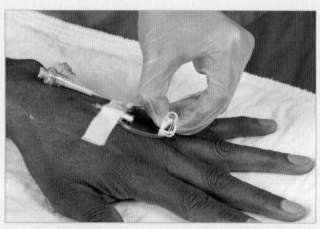

FIGURE 5. Clamping the access port. *(Photo by B. Proud.)*

27. Discard the syringe in the appropriate receptacle.

 28. Remove PPE, if used. Perform hand hygiene.

29. Document the administration of the medication immediately after administration. See Documentation section below.

30. Evaluate the patient's response to medication within appropriate time frame.

31. Check the medication lock site at least every 8 hours or according to facility policy.

Proper disposal prevents injury.

Removing PPE properly reduces the risk for infection transmission and contamination of other items. Hand hygiene prevents the spread of microorganisms.

Timely documentation helps to ensure patient safety.

The patient needs to be evaluated for therapeutic and adverse effects from the medication.

This ensures patency of system.

EVALUATION

The expected outcomes are met when the medication is delivered via the intravenous route using sterile technique; the medication is delivered to the patient in a safe manner and at the appropriate infusion rate; patient experiences no adverse effect; the intermittent peripheral venous access device remains patent; and the patient understands and complies with the medication regimen.

DOCUMENTATION

Guidelines

Document the administration of the medication and/or saline flush, including date, time, dose, route of administration, site of administration, and rate of administration on the CMAR/MAR or record using the required format, immediately after administration. If using a bar-code system, medication administration is automatically recorded when the bar code is scanned. PRN medications require documentation of the reason for administration. Prompt recording avoids the possibility of accidentally repeating the administration of the drug. If the drug was refused or omitted, record this in the appropriate area on the medication record and notify the primary care provider. This verifies the reason medication was omitted and ensures that the primary care provider is aware of the patient's condition.

UNEXPECTED SITUATIONS AND ASSOCIATED INTERVENTIONS

- *Upon assessing the medication lock site before administering medication, you note that the medication lock has infiltrated:* Remove medication lock from extremity. Restart peripheral venous access in a different location. Continue to monitor new site as medication is administered.
- *While you are administering medication, patient begins to complain of pain at the site:* Stop the medication. Assess the medication lock site for signs of infiltration and phlebitis. Flush the medication lock with normal saline again to recheck patency. If the IV site appears within normal limits, resume medication administration at a slower rate. If pain persists, stop, remove medication lock and restart in a different location.
- *As you are attempting to access lock, tip of syringe touches patient's arm:* Discard syringe. Prepare a new dose for administration.
- *No blood return is noted upon aspiration:* If medication lock appears patent, without signs of infiltration, and normal saline fluid infuses without difficulty, proceed with administration. Observe closely for signs and symptoms of infiltration during and after administration.

SPECIAL CONSIDERATIONS

General Considerations

- If medication lock is not used, flush with saline every 8 to 12 hours to maintain patency, according to facility policy.
- Routinely change the medication lock site every 72 to 96 hours, according to facility policy. This reduces the risk of infection and emboli in the bloodstream.
- Intermittent infusions of small-volume IV medications can also be administered through the medication lock. Attach IV medication container to infusion tubing and prime. After flushing the medication lock with saline as outlined above, attach the infusion tubing to the medication lock. Adjust infusion rate with roller clamp on infusion tubing. After infusion is completed, remove tubing from lock and flush with saline as outlined above.
- Ongoing assessment is an important part of nursing care to evaluate patient response to administered medications and early detection of adverse effects. If an adverse effect is suspected, withhold further medication doses and notify the patient's primary healthcare provider. Additional intervention is based on type of reaction and patient assessment.

Infant and Child Considerations

- If the volume of medication being administered is small (less than 1.0 mL), always include the amount of flush solution as part of the total amount to be injected and take this into account when determining how fast to push a medication. For example, if the medication is to be injected at a rate of 1.0 mL per minute and the total amount of solution to be injected is 2.25 mL (0.25 mL medication volume plus 2.0 mL saline flush solution volume equals 2.25 mL), then the medication would be injected over a period of 2 minutes 15 seconds.

Skill · 15   Instilling Eye Drops

Eye drops are instilled for their local effects, such as for pupil dilation or constriction when examining the eye, for infection treatment, or for controlling intraocular pressure (for patients with glaucoma). The type and amount of solution depend on the purpose of the instillation.

The eye is a delicate organ, highly susceptible to infection and injury. Although the eye is never free of microorganisms, the secretions of the conjunctiva protect against many pathogens. For maximal safety for the patient, the equipment, solutions, and ointments introduced into the conjunctival sac should be sterile. If this is not possible, follow careful guidelines for medical asepsis.

Refer to the accompanying Skill Variation for the steps to administer eye ointment.

(continued)

Skill · 15   Instilling Eye Drops   *continued*

EQUIPMENT

- Gloves
- Additional PPE, as indicated
- Medication
- Tissues
- Normal saline solution
- Washcloth, cotton balls, or gauze squares
- Computer-generated Medication Administration Record (CMAR) or Medication Administration Record (MAR)

ASSESSMENT

Assess the patient for any allergies. Check the expiration date before administering medication. Assess the appropriateness of the drug for the patient. Review assessment and laboratory data that may influence drug administration. Verify patient name, dose, route, and time of administration. Assess the affected eye for any drainage, erythema, or swelling. Assess the patient's knowledge of the medication. If the patient has a knowledge deficit about the medication, this may be the appropriate time to begin education about the medication. If the medication may affect the patient's vital signs, assess them before administration.

NURSING DIAGNOSIS

Determine related factors for the nursing diagnoses based on the patient's current status. Appropriate nursing diagnoses may include:

- Risk for Allergy Response
- Deficient Knowledge
- Risk for Injury

OUTCOME IDENTIFICATION AND PLANNING

The expected outcome to achieve when administering eye drops is that the medication is delivered successfully into the eye. Other outcomes that may be appropriate include the following: patient experiences no allergy response; patient does not exhibit systemic effects of the medication; patient's eye remains free from injury; and patient understands the rationale for medication administration.

IMPLEMENTATION

ACTION	RATIONALE
1. Gather equipment. Check medication order against the original order in the medical record, according to facility policy. Clarify any inconsistencies. Check the patient's chart for allergies.	This comparison helps to identify errors that may have occurred when orders were transcribed. The primary care provider's order is the legal record of medication orders for each facility.
2. Know the actions, special nursing considerations, safe dose ranges, purpose of administration, and adverse effects of the medications to be administered. Consider the appropriateness of the medication for this patient.	This knowledge aids the nurse in evaluating the therapeutic effect of the medication in relation to the patient's disorder and can also be used to educate the patient about the medication.
3. Perform hand hygiene.	Hand hygiene prevents the spread of microorganisms.
4. Move the medication cart to the outside of the patient's room or prepare for administration in the medication area.	Organization facilitates error-free administration and saves time.
5. Unlock the medication cart or drawer. Enter pass code and scan employee identification, if required.	Locking the cart or drawer safeguards each patient's medication supply. Hospital accrediting organizations require medication carts to be locked when not in use. Entering pass code and scanning ID allows only authorized users into the system and identifies user for documentation by the computer.
6. **Prepare medications for one patient at a time.**	This prevents errors in medication administration.
7. Read the CMAR/MAR and select the proper medication from the patient's medication drawer or unit stock.	This is the *first* check of the label.
8. Compare the label with the CMAR/MAR. Check expiration dates and perform calculations, if necessary. Scan the bar code on the package, if required.	This is the *second* check of the label. Verify calculations with another nurse to ensure safety, if necessary.

ACTION

RATIONALE

9. **When all medications for one patient have been prepared, recheck the label with the CMAR/MAR before taking them to the patient.**

This is a *third* check to ensure accuracy and to prevent errors. Some facilities require the third check to occur at the bedside, after identifying the patient and before administration.

10. Lock the medication cart before leaving it.

Locking the cart or drawer safeguards the patient's medication supply. Hospital accrediting organizations require medication carts to be locked when not in use.

11. Transport medications to the patient's bedside carefully, and keep the medications in sight at all times.

Careful handling and close observation prevent accidental or deliberate disarrangement of medications.

12. **Ensure that the patient receives the medications at the correct time.**

Check agency policy, which may allow for administration within a period of 30 minutes before or 30 minutes after designated time.

13. Perform hand hygiene and put on PPE, if indicated.

Hand hygiene and PPE prevent the spread of microorganisms. PPE is required based on transmission precautions.

14. Identify the patient. Usually, the patient should be identified using two methods. Compare information with the CMAR/MAR.

Identifying the patient ensures the right patient receives the medications and helps prevent errors.

a. Check the name and identification number on the patient's identification band.

This is the most reliable method. Replace the identification band if it is missing or inaccurate in any way.

b. Ask the patient to state his or her name and birth date, based on facility policy.

This requires a response from the patient, but illness and strange surroundings often cause patients to be confused.

c. If the patient cannot identify him- or herself, verify the patient's identification with a staff member who knows the patient for the second source.

This is another way to double-check identity. Do not use the name on the door or over the bed, because these signs may be inaccurate.

15. Complete necessary assessments before administering medications. Check the patient's allergy bracelet or ask the patient about allergies. Explain the purpose and action of each medication to the patient.

Assessment is a prerequisite to administration of medications.

16. Scan the patient's bar code on the identification band, if required.

Provides an additional check to ensure that the medication is given to the right patient.

17. Put on gloves.

Gloves protect the nurse from potential contact with mucous membranes and body fluids.

18. Offer tissue to patient.

Solution and tears may spill from the eye during the procedure.

19. Cleanse the eyelids and eyelashes of any drainage with a washcloth, cotton balls, or gauze squares moistened with normal saline solution. Use each area of the cleaning surface once, moving from the inner toward the outer canthus (Figure 1).

Debris can be carried into the eye when the conjunctival sac is exposed. Using each area of the gauze once and moving from the inner canthus to the outer canthus prevents carrying debris to the lacrimal ducts.

20. Tilt the patient's head back slightly if sitting, or place the patient's head over a pillow if lying down. The head may be turned slightly to the affected side to prevent solution or tears from flowing toward the opposite eye (Figure 2).

Tilting patient's head back slightly makes it easier to reach the conjunctival sac. This should be avoided if the patient has a cervical spine injury. Turning the head to the affected side helps to prevent solution or tears from flowing toward the opposite eye.

21. Remove the cap from the medication bottle, being careful not to touch the inner side of the cap. (See the accompanying Skill Variation for administering ointment.)

Touching the inner side of the cap may contaminate the bottle of medication.

22. Invert the monodrip plastic container that is commonly used to instill eye drops. Have patient look up and focus on something on the ceiling.

By having the patient look up and focus on something else, the procedure is less traumatic and keeps the eye still.

(continued)

Skill · 15 **Instilling Eye Drops** *continued*

ACTION

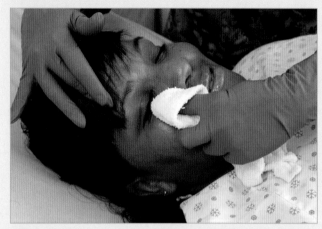

FIGURE 1. Cleaning lids and lashes from inside of eye to outside.

23. Place thumb or two fingers near margin of lower eyelid immediately below eyelashes, and exert pressure downward over bony prominence of cheek. Lower conjunctival sac is exposed as lower lid is pulled down (Figure 3).

24. **Hold dropper close to eye, but avoid touching eyelids or lashes.** Squeeze container and allow prescribed number of drops to fall in lower conjunctival sac (Figure 4).

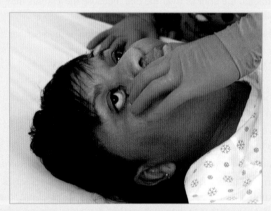

FIGURE 3. Exerting pressure downward to expose lower conjunctival sac.

25. Release lower lid after eye drops are instilled. Ask patient to close eyes gently.

26. Apply gentle pressure over inner canthus to prevent eye drops from flowing into tear duct (Figure 5).

27. Instruct patient not to rub affected eye.

28. Remove gloves. Assist patient to a comfortable position.

 29. Remove additional PPE, if used. Perform hand hygiene.

RATIONALE

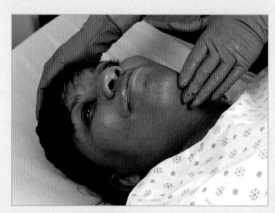

FIGURE 2. Turning head slightly to affected side.

The eye drop should be placed in the conjunctival sac, not directly on the eyeball.

Touching the eye, eyelids, or lashes can contaminate the medication in the bottle; startle the patient, causing blinking; or injure the eye. Do not allow medication to fall onto cornea. This may injure the cornea or cause the patient to have an unpleasant sensation.

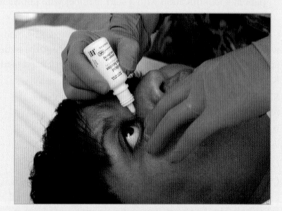

FIGURE 4. Administering drops into conjunctival sac.

This allows the medication to be distributed over the entire eye.

This minimizes the risk of systemic effects from the medication.

This prevents injury and irritation to eye.

This ensures patient comfort.

Removing PPE properly reduces the risk for infection transmission and contamination of other items. Hand hygiene prevents the spread of microorganisms.

ACTION

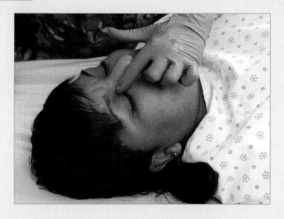

FIGURE 5. Applying gentle pressure over inner canthus.

RATIONALE

30. Document the administration of the medication immediately after administration. See Documentation section below.

Timely documentation helps to ensure patient safety.

31. Evaluate the patient's response to medication within appropriate time frame.

The patient needs to be evaluated for therapeutic and adverse effects from the medication.

EVALUATION

The expected outcomes are met when the patient receives the eye drops; experiences no adverse effects, including allergy response, systemic effect, or injury; and understands the rationale for the medication administration.

DOCUMENTATION
Guidelines

Document the administration of the medication immediately after administration, including date, time, dose, route of administration, and site of administration, specifically right, left, or both eyes, on the CMAR/MAR or record using the required format. If using a bar-code system, medication administration is automatically recorded when the bar code is scanned. PRN medications require documentation of the reason for administration. Prompt recording avoids the possibility of accidentally repeating the administration of the drug. If the drug was refused or omitted, record this in the appropriate area on the medication record and notify the primary care provider. This verifies the reason medication was omitted and ensures that the primary care provider is aware of the patient's condition.

UNEXPECTED SITUATIONS AND ASSOCIATED INTERVENTIONS

- *Drop is placed on eyelid or outer margin of eyelid due to patient blinking or moving:* Do not count this drop in total number of drops administered. Allow the patient to regain composure and proceed with application of medication. Consider approaching the patient from below the line of sight.
- *You cannot open eyelids due to dried crust and matting of eyelids:* Place a warm, wet washcloth over the eye and allow it to remain there for approximately 3 minutes. Cleanse eye as described previously. You may need to repeat this procedure if there is a large amount of matting.
- *Bottle or tube of medication comes in contact with eyeball when applying medication:* Bottle is contaminated; discard appropriately. Notify pharmacy or retrieve a new bottle for the oncoming shift.

SPECIAL CONSIDERATIONS
General Considerations

- Ongoing assessment is an important part of nursing care to evaluate patient response to administered medications and early detection of adverse effects. If an adverse effect is suspected, withhold further medication doses and notify the patient's primary healthcare provider. Additional intervention is based on type of reaction and patient assessment.

Infant and Child Considerations

- To apply eye drops in a small child, two or more people may be needed to restrain the child. Make sure the child does not reach up to the eye for fear of jabbing the medication bottle into the eye.

(continued)

Skill · 15   Instilling Eye Drops   *continued*

Skill Variation   Administering Eye Ointment

1. Check medication order against the original order in the medical record, according to facility policy. Clarify any inconsistencies. Check the patient's chart for allergies. Know the actions, special nursing considerations, safe dose ranges, purpose of administration, and adverse effects of the medications to be administered. Consider the appropriateness of the medication for this patient.

2. Perform hand hygiene.

3. Move the medication cart to the outside of the patient's room or prepare for administration in the medication area.

4. Unlock the medication cart or drawer. Enter pass code and scan employee identification, if required.

5. Read the CMAR/MAR and select the proper medication from the patient's medication drawer or unit stock.

6. Compare the label with the CMAR/MAR. Check expiration dates. Scan the bar code on the package, if required.

7. When all medications for one patient have been prepared, recheck the label with the CMAR/MAR before taking it to the patient. Some facilities require the third check to occur at the bedside, after identifying the patient and before administration.

8. Lock the medication cart before leaving it.

9. Transport medications and equipment to the patient's bedside carefully, and keep the medications in sight at all times.

10. Perform hand hygiene and put on PPE, if indicated.

11. Identify the patient. The patient should be identified using two methods.

12. Close the door to the room or pull the bedside curtain.

13. Complete necessary assessments before administering medications. Check allergy bracelet or ask patient about allergies. Explain the purpose and action of the medication to the patient.

14. Scan the patient's bar code on the identification band, if required.

15. Put on gloves. Offer the patient a tissue.

16. Cleanse the eyelids and eyelashes of any drainage with cotton balls or gauze squares moistened with normal saline solution. Use each area of the gauze square once, moving from the inner toward the outer canthus.

17. Tilt the patient's head back slightly if sitting, or place the patient's head over a pillow if lying down. The head may be turned slightly to the affected side to prevent solution or tears from flowing toward the opposite eye.

18. Have patient look up and focus on something on the ceiling.

19. Place thumb or two fingers near margin of lower eyelid immediately below eyelashes and exert pressure downward over bony prominence of cheek. Lower conjunctival sac is exposed as lower lid is pulled down.

20. Hold the ointment tube close to eye, but avoid touching eyelids or lashes. Squeeze container and apply about ½ inch of ointment from the tube along the exposed sac. Apply the medication moving from the inner canthus to the outer canthus. Twist tube to break off ribbon of ointment. Do not touch the tip to the eye.

21. Release lower lid after ointment is instilled. Ask patient to close eyes gently.

22. The warmth helps to liquefy the ointment. Instruct the patient to move the eye, because this helps to spread the ointment under the lids and over the surface of the eyeball.

23. Assist the patient to a comfortable position. Explain that the ointment may temporarily blur vision; encourage the patient not to rub the eye.

24. Remove gloves and additional PPE, if used. Perform hand hygiene.

25. Document administration of the medication on the CMAR/MAR immediately after administering the medication.

26. Evaluate the patient's response to medication within appropriate time frame.

Skill · 16   Instilling Ear Drops

Drugs are instilled into the auditory canal for their local effect. They are used to soften wax, relieve pain, apply local anesthesia, and treat infections.

The tympanic membrane separates the external ear from the middle ear. Normally, it is intact and closes the entrance to the middle ear completely. If it is ruptured or has been opened by surgical intervention, the middle ear and the inner ear have a direct passage to the external ear. When this occurs, perform installations with the greatest of care to prevent forcing materials from the outer ear into the middle ear and the inner ear. Use sterile technique to prevent infection.

EQUIPMENT

- Medication (warmed to 37°C [98.6°F])
- Dropper
- Tissue
- Cotton ball (optional)
- Gloves
- Additional PPE, as indicated
- Washcloth (optional)
- Normal saline solution
- Computer-generated Medication Administration Record (CMAR) or Medication Administration Record (MAR)

ASSESSMENT

Assess the affected ear for redness, erythema, edema, drainage, or tenderness. Assess the patient for allergies. Verify patient name, dose, route, and time of administration. Assess the patient's knowledge of medication and procedure. If the patient has a knowledge deficit about the medication, this may be an appropriate time to begin education about the medication. Assess the patient's ability to cooperate with the procedure.

NURSING DIAGNOSIS

Determine related factors for the nursing diagnoses based on the patient's current status. Appropriate nursing diagnoses may include:

- Deficient Knowledge
- Anxiety
- Risk for Injury
- Acute Pain
- Risk for Allergy Response

OUTCOME IDENTIFICATION AND PLANNING

The expected outcome to achieve is that drops are administered successfully. Other outcomes that may be appropriate include the following: patient understands the rationale for the ear drop installation and has decreased anxiety; patient remains free from pain; and patient experiences no allergy response or injury.

IMPLEMENTATION

ACTION	RATIONALE
1. Gather equipment. Check medication order against the original order in the medical record, according to facility policy. Clarify any inconsistencies. Check the patient's chart for allergies.	This comparison helps to identify errors that may have occurred when orders were transcribed. The primary care provider's order is the legal record of medication orders for each facility.
2. Know the actions, special nursing considerations, safe dose ranges, purpose of administration, and adverse effects of the medication to be administered. Consider the appropriateness of the medication for this patient.	This knowledge aids the nurse in evaluating the therapeutic effect of the medication in relation to the patient's disorder and can also be used to educate the patient about the medication.
3. Perform hand hygiene.	Hand hygiene prevents the spread of microorganisms.
4. Move the medication cart to the outside of the patient's room or prepare for administration in the medication area.	Organization facilitates error-free administration and saves time.

(continued)

Skill · 16   Instilling Ear Drops   *continued*

ACTION	RATIONALE
5. Unlock the medication cart or drawer. Enter pass code and scan employee identification, if required.	Locking the cart or drawer safeguards each patient's medication supply. Hospital accrediting organizations require medication carts to be locked when not in use. Entering pass code and scanning ID allows only authorized users into the system and identifies user for documentation by the computer.
6. **Prepare medications for one patient at a time.**	This prevents errors in medication administration.
7. Read the CMAR/MAR and select the proper medication from the patient's medication drawer or unit stock.	This is the *first* check of the label.
8. Compare the label with the CMAR/MAR. Check expiration dates and perform calculations, if necessary. Scan the bar code on the package, if required.	This is the *second* check of the label. Verify calculations with another nurse to ensure safety, if necessary.
9. **When all medications for one patient have been prepared, recheck the label with the CMAR/MAR before taking them to the patient.**	This is a *third* check to ensure accuracy and to prevent errors. Some facilities require the third check to occur at the bedside, after identifying the patient and before administration.
10. Lock the medication cart before leaving it.	Locking the cart or drawer safeguards the patient's medication supply. Hospital accrediting organizations require medication carts to be locked when not in use.
11. Transport medications to the patient's bedside carefully, and keep the medications in sight at all times.	Careful handling and close observation prevent accidental or deliberate disarrangement of medications.
12. **Ensure that the patient receives the medications at the correct time.**	Check agency policy, which may allow for administration within a period of 30 minutes before or 30 minutes after designated time.
13. Perform hand hygiene and put on PPE, if indicated.	Hand hygiene and PPE prevent the spread of microorganisms. PPE is required based on transmission precautions.
14. Identify the patient. Usually, the patient should be identified using two methods. Compare information with the CMAR/MAR.	Identifying the patient ensures the right patient receives the medications and helps prevent errors.
a. Check the name and identification number on the patient's identification band.	This is the most reliable method. Replace the identification band if it is missing or inaccurate in any way.
b. Ask the patient to state his or her name and birth date, based on facility policy.	This requires a response from the patient, but illness and strange surroundings often cause patients to be confused.
c. If the patient cannot identify him- or herself, verify the patient's identification with a staff member who knows the patient for the second source.	This is another way to double-check identity. Do not use the name on the door or over the bed, because these signs may be inaccurate.
15. Complete necessary assessments before administering medications. Check the patient's allergy bracelet or ask the patient about allergies. Explain the purpose and action of each medication to the patient.	Assessment is a prerequisite to administration of medications.
16. Scan the patient's bar code on the identification band, if required.	Provides an additional check to ensure that the medication is given to the right patient.
17. Put on gloves.	Gloves protect the nurse from potential contact with contaminants and body fluids.
18. Cleanse external ear of any drainage with cotton ball or washcloth moistened with normal saline (Figure 1).	Debris and drainage may prevent some of the medication from entering the ear canal.
19. Place patient on his or her unaffected side in bed, or, if ambulatory, have patient sit with head well tilted to the side so that affected ear is uppermost (Figure 2).	This positioning prevents the drops from escaping from the ear.

ACTION

20. Draw up the amount of solution needed in the dropper. Do not return excess medication to stock bottle. A prepackaged, monodrip plastic container may also be used (Figure 3).

21. Straighten auditory canal by pulling cartilaginous portion of pinna up and back for an adult.

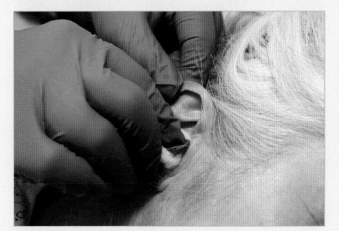

FIGURE 1. Cleaning external ear.

22. Hold dropper in the ear with its tip above the auditory canal (Figure 4). Do not touch the dropper to the ear. For an infant or an irrational or confused patient, protect the dropper with a piece of soft tubing to help prevent injury to the ear.

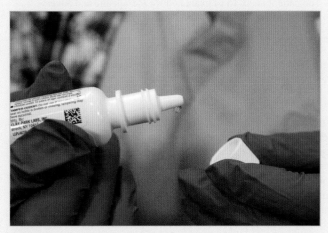

FIGURE 3. Prepackaged ear drop solution.

23. **Allow drops to fall on the side of the canal.**

24. Release pinna after instilling drops, and have patient maintain the position to prevent escape of medication.

25. Gently press on the tragus a few times (Figure 5).

RATIONALE

Risk for contamination is increased when medication is returned to the stock bottle.

Pulling on the pinna as described helps to straighten the canal properly for ear drop instillation.

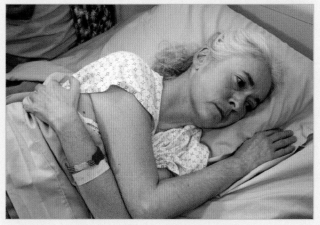

FIGURE 2. Positioning patient on unaffected side.

By holding the dropper in the ear, most of the medication will enter the ear canal. Touching the dropper to the ear contaminates the dropper and medication. The hard tip of the dropper can damage the tympanic membrane if it is jabbed into the ear.

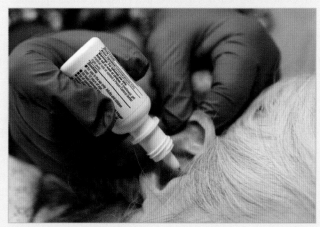

FIGURE 4. Pulling the pinna up and back and placing the tip of dropper above auditory canal.

It is uncomfortable for the patient if the drops fall directly onto the tympanic membrane.

Medication should remain in ear canal for at least 5 minutes.

Pressing on the tragus causes medication from the canal to move toward the tympanic membrane.

(continued)

Skill · 16 **Instilling Ear Drops** *continued*

ACTION

26. If ordered, loosely insert a cotton ball into the ear canal (Figure 6).

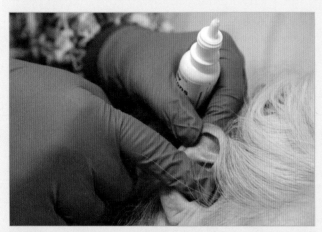

FIGURE 5. Applying pressure to tragus.

27. Remove gloves. Assist the patient to a comfortable position.

 28. Remove additional PPE, if used. Perform hand hygiene.

29. Document the administration of the medication immediately after administration. See Documentation section below.

30. Evaluate the patient's response to medication within appropriate time frame.

RATIONALE

A cotton ball can help prevent medication from leaking out of ear canal.

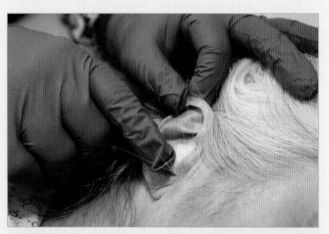

FIGURE 6. Inserting cotton ball into ear canal.

This ensures patient comfort.

Removing PPE properly reduces the risk for infection transmission and contamination of other items. Hand hygiene prevents the spread of microorganisms.

Timely documentation helps to ensure patient safety.

The patient needs to be evaluated for therapeutic and adverse effects from the medication.

EVALUATION

The expected outcomes are met when the patient receives the ear drops successfully; understands the rationale for ear drop instillation and exhibits no or decreased anxiety; experiences no or minimal pain; and experiences no allergy response or injury.

DOCUMENTATION
Guidelines

Document the administration of the medication immediately after administration, including date, time, dose, route of administration, and site of administration, specifically right, left, or both ears, on the CMAR/MAR or record using the required format. If using a bar-code system, medication administration is automatically recorded when the bar code is scanned. PRN medications require documentation of the reason for administration. Prompt recording avoids the possibility of accidentally repeating the administration of the drug. Document pre- and postadministration assessments, characteristics of any drainage, and the patient's response to the treatment, if appropriate. If the drug was refused or omitted, record this in the appropriate area on the medication record and notify the primary care provider. This verifies the reason medication was omitted and ensures that the primary care provider is aware of the patient's condition.

UNEXPECTED SITUATIONS AND ASSOCIATED INTERVENTIONS

- *Medication runs from ear into eye:* Notify primary care provider and check with the pharmacy. Eye irrigation may need to be performed.
- *Patient complains of extreme pain when you press on the tragus:* Allow patient to press on tragus. If pressure causes too much pain, this part may be deferred.

SPECIAL CONSIDERATIONS

General Considerations

- If both ears are to be treated, wait 5 minutes before instilling drops into the second ear.
- Ongoing assessment is an important part of nursing care to evaluate patient response to administered treatments and early detection of adverse effects. If an adverse effect is suspected, notify the patient's primary healthcare provider. Additional intervention is based on type of reaction and patient assessment.

Infant and Child Considerations

- Pull pinna straight back for a child older than 3 years (Figure 7) and down and back for an infant or a child younger than 3 years (Figure 8).
- Distraction techniques, such as TV or a quiet toy, may be helpful when attempting to keep a child quiet for 5 minutes. Reading to the child may not be appropriate because the child's hearing may be compromised during medication administration.

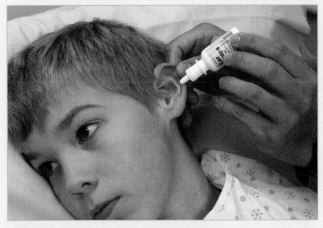

FIGURE 7. Pulling pinna straight back for child older than 3 years.

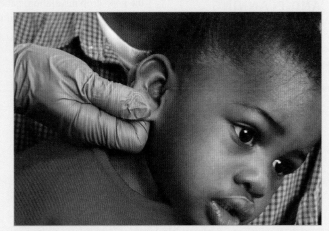

FIGURE 8. Pulling pinna down and back for an infant or child younger than 3 years.

Skill · 17   Instilling Nose Drops

Nasal instillations are used to treat allergies, sinus infections, and nasal congestion. Medications with a systemic effect, such as vasopressin, may also be prepared as a nasal instillation. The nose is normally not a sterile cavity, but because of its connection with the sinuses, it is important to observe medical asepsis carefully when using nasal instillations.

The following skill describes the steps to administer nasal drops. Refer to the accompanying Skill Variation for guidelines to administer medication via a nasal spray.

EQUIPMENT

- Medication
- Dropper, if not part of medication container
- Gloves
- Additional PPE, as indicated
- Tissue
- Computer-generated Medication Administration Record (CMAR) or Medication Administration Record (MAR)

(continued)

Skill · 17   Instilling Nose Drops   *continued*

ASSESSMENT

Assess the nares for redness, erythema, edema, drainage, or tenderness. Assess the patient for allergies. Verify patient name, dose, route, and time of administration. Assess the patient's knowledge of medication and procedure. If the patient has a knowledge deficit about the medication, this may be an appropriate time to begin education about the procedure. Assess the patient's ability to cooperate with the procedure.

NURSING DIAGNOSIS

Determine related factors for the nursing diagnoses based on the patient's current status. Appropriate nursing diagnoses may include:
- Deficient Knowledge
- Risk for Allergy Response

OUTCOME IDENTIFICATION AND PLANNING

The expected outcome to achieve is that the medication is administered successfully into the nose. Other outcomes that may be appropriate include the following: patient understands the rationale for the nose-drop instillation; patient experiences no allergy response; patient's skin remains intact; patient experiences no, or minimal, pain.

IMPLEMENTATION

ACTION

1. Gather equipment. Check medication order against the original order in the medical record, according to facility policy. Clarify any inconsistencies. Check the patient's chart for allergies.

2. Know the actions, special nursing considerations, safe dose ranges, purpose of administration, and adverse effects of the medication to be administered. Consider the appropriateness of the medication for this patient.

      3. Perform hand hygiene.

4. Move the medication cart to the outside of the patient's room or prepare for administration in the medication area.

5. Unlock the medication cart or drawer. Enter pass code and scan employee identification, if required.

6. **Prepare medications for one patient at a time.**

7. Read the CMAR/MAR and select the proper medication from the patient's medication drawer or unit stock.

8. Compare the label with the CMAR/MAR. Check expiration dates and perform calculations, if necessary. Scan the bar code on the package, if required.

9. **When all medications for one patient have been prepared, recheck the label with the CMAR/MAR before taking them to the patient.**

10. Lock the medication cart before leaving it.

11. Transport medications to the patient's bedside carefully, and keep the medications in sight at all times.

12. **Ensure that the patient receives the medications at the correct time.**

RATIONALE

This comparison helps to identify errors that may have occurred when orders were transcribed. The primary care provider's order is the legal record of medication orders for each facility.

This knowledge aids the nurse in evaluating the therapeutic effect of the medication in relation to the patient's disorder and can also be used to educate the patient about the medication.

Hand hygiene prevents the spread of microorganisms.

Organization facilitates error-free administration and saves time.

Locking the cart or drawer safeguards each patient's medication supply. Hospital accrediting organizations require medication carts to be locked when not in use. Entering pass code and scanning ID allows only authorized users into the system and identifies user for documentation by the computer.

This prevents errors in medication administration.

This is the *first* check of the label.

This is the *second* check of the label. Verify calculations with another nurse to ensure safety, if necessary.

This is a *third* check to ensure accuracy and to prevent errors. Some facilities require the third check to occur at the bedside, after identifying the patient and before administration.

Locking the cart or drawer safeguards the patient's medication supply. Hospital accrediting organizations require medication carts to be locked when not in use.

Careful handling and close observation prevent accidental or deliberate disarrangement of medications.

Check agency policy, which may allow for administration within a period of 30 minutes before or 30 minutes after designated time.

ACTION

13. Perform hand hygiene and put on PPE, if indicated.

14. Identify the patient. Usually, the patient should be identified using two methods. Compare information with the CMAR/MAR.

   a. Check the name and identification number on the patient's identification band.

   b. Ask the patient to state his or her name and birth date, based on facility policy.

   c. If the patient cannot identify him- or herself, verify the patient's identification with a staff member who knows the patient for the second source.

15. Complete necessary assessments before administering medications. Check the patient's allergy bracelet or ask the patient about allergies. Explain the purpose and action of each medication to the patient.

16. Scan the patient's bar code on the identification band, if required.

17. Put on gloves.

18. Provide patient with paper tissues and ask patient to blow his or her nose.

19. Have patient sit up with head tilted well back. If patient is lying down, tilt head back over a pillow (Figure 1).

20. Draw sufficient solution into dropper for both nares. Do not return excess solution to a stock bottle.

21. Ask the patient to breathe through the mouth. Hold tip of nose up and place dropper just above naris, about ⅓ inch (Figure 2). Instill the prescribed number of drops in one naris and then into the other. Protect dropper with a piece of soft tubing if patient is an infant or young child. Avoid touching naris with dropper.

RATIONALE

Hand hygiene and PPE prevent the spread of microorganisms. PPE is required based on transmission precautions.

Identifying the patient ensures the right patient receives the medications and helps prevent errors.

This is the most reliable method. Replace the identification band if it is missing or inaccurate in any way.

This requires a response from the patient, but illness and strange surroundings often cause patients to be confused.

This is another way to double-check identity. Do not use the name on the door or over the bed, because these signs may be inaccurate.

Assessment is a prerequisite to administration of medications.

Provides an additional check to ensure that the medication is given to the right patient.

Gloves protect the nurse from potential contact with contaminants and body fluids.

Blowing the nose clears the nasal mucosa prior to medication administration.

These positions allow the solution to flow well back into the nares. Do not tilt the head if patient has a cervical spine injury.

Returning solution to a stock bottle increases the risk for contamination of the stock bottle.

Breathing through the mouth helps prevent aspiration of solution. The soft tubing will protect the patient's nares from injury during administration of medication. Touching the naris may cause the patient to sneeze and will contaminate the dropper.

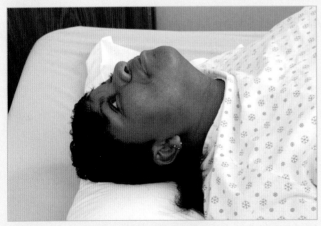

FIGURE 1. Patient lying down, head tilted back over pillow.

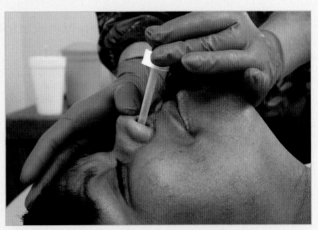

FIGURE 2. Positioning nose dropper just above naris, about ⅓ of an inch.

(continued)

Skill · 17   Instilling Nose Drops   *continued*

ACTION	RATIONALE
22. Have patient remain in position with head tilted back for a few minutes.	Tilting the head back prevents the escape of the medication.
23. Remove gloves. Assist the patient to a comfortable position.	This ensures patient comfort.
24. Remove additional PPE, if used. Perform hand hygiene.	Removing PPE properly reduces the risk for infection transmission and contamination of other items. Hand hygiene prevents the spread of microorganisms.
25. Document the administration of the medication immediately after administration. See Documentation section below.	Timely documentation helps to ensure patient safety.
26. Evaluate the patient's response to the procedure and medication within appropriate time frame.	The patient needs to be evaluated for therapeutic and adverse effects from the medication.

EVALUATION   The expected outcomes are met when the patient receives the nose drops successfully; understands the rationale for nose-drop instillation; and experiences no allergy response; patient's skin remains intact; and patient experiences no, or minimal, pain or discomfort.

DOCUMENTATION
Guidelines

Document the administration of the medication, including date, time, dose, route of administration, and site of administration, specifically right, left, or both nares, on the CMAR/MAR or record using the required format. If using a bar-code system, medication administration is automatically recorded when the bar code is scanned. PRN medications require documentation of the reason for administration. Prompt recording avoids the possibility of accidentally repeating the administration of the drug. Document pre- and postadministration assessments, characteristics of any drainage, and the patient's response to the treatment, if appropriate. If the drug was refused or omitted, record this in the appropriate area on the medication record and notify the primary care provider. This verifies the reason medication was omitted and ensures that the primary care provider is aware of the patient's condition.

UNEXPECTED SITUATIONS AND ASSOCIATED INTERVENTIONS

• *Patient sneezes immediately after receiving nose drops:* Do not repeat the dosage, because you cannot determine how much medication was actually absorbed.

SPECIAL CONSIDERATIONS

• Ongoing assessment is an important part of nursing care to evaluate patient response to administered medications and early detection of adverse effects. If an adverse effect is suspected, withhold further medication doses and notify the patient's primary healthcare provider. Additional intervention is based on type of reaction and patient assessment.

Skill Variation   Administering Medication via Nasal Spray

1. Check medication order against the original order in the medical record, according to facility policy. Clarify any inconsistencies. Check the patient's chart for allergies. Know the actions, special nursing considerations, safe dose ranges, purpose of administration, and adverse effects of the medications to be administered. Consider the appropriateness of the medication for this patient.

 2. Perform hand hygiene.

3. Move the medication cart to the outside of the patient's room or prepare for administration in the medication area.

4. Unlock the medication cart or drawer. Enter pass code and scan employee identification, if required.

5. Read the CMAR/MAR and select the proper medication from the patient's medication drawer or unit stock.

6. Compare the label with the CMAR/MAR. Check expiration dates. Scan the bar code on the package, if required.

7. When all medications for one patient have been prepared, recheck the label with the CMAR/MAR before taking it to the patient. Some facilities require the third check to occur at the bedside, after identifying the patient and before administration.

8. Lock the medication cart before leaving it.

Skill Variation Administering Medication via Nasal Spray *continued*

9. Transport medications and equipment to the patient's bedside carefully, and keep the medications in sight at all times.

10. Perform hand hygiene and put on PPE, if indicated.

11. Identify the patient. The patient should be identified using two methods.

12. Close the door to the room or pull the bedside curtain.

13. Complete necessary assessments before administering medications. Check allergy bracelet or ask patient about allergies. Explain the purpose and action of the medication to the patient.

14. Scan the patient's bar code on the identification band, if required.

15. Put on gloves. Assist the patient to an upright position with the head tilted back.

16. Instruct the patient to inhale gently through the nose as the spray is being administered.

17. Have the patient hold one nostril closed. If the spray is indicated for only one naris, close the nostril that will not receive the medication.

18. Agitate the medication container, if required, to mix the contents thoroughly.

19. Insert the nozzle of the medication container just into the nostril.

20. Compress the container, spraying the medication into the nostril, while the patient gently inhales through the nostril.

21. Keep the medication container compressed and remove from the nostril. Release the container from the compressed state. Do not allow the container to return to its original position until it is removed from the patient's nose to prevent contamination of the contents of the container.

22. Repeat in the other nostril, if prescribed.

23. Instruct the patient to maintain head position for 1 to 2 minutes.

24. Remove gloves. Assist the patient to a comfortable position.

25. Remove additional PPE, if used. Perform hand hygiene.

26. Document administration of the medication on the CMAR/MAR immediately after administering the medication. Document the site, if only one nostril is used.

27. Evaluate the patient's response to medication within appropriate time frame.